Geilton Xavier Matos

Antimicrobial activity of Miconia ligustroides

Geilton Xavier Matos

Antimicrobial activity of Miconia ligustroides

Isolation of Acid Triterpenes from Miconia L., Preparation of Derivatives and Evaluation of Antimicrobial Activity

ScienciaScripts

Imprint

Cover image: www.ingimage.com

This book is a translation from the original published under ISBN 978-3-330-76743-0.

Publisher:
Sciencia Scripts
is a trademark of
Dodo Books Indian Ocean Ltd. and OmniScriptum S.R.L publishing group

120 High Road, East Finchley, London, N2 9ED, United Kingdom
Str. Armeneasca 28/1, office 1, Chisinau MD-2012, Republic of Moldova, Europe
Managing Directors: Ieva Konstantinova, Victoria Ursu
info@omniscriptum.com

Printed at: see last page
ISBN: 978-620-8-57690-5

SUMMARY

SUMMARY

The present study reports phytochemical studies and evaluation of the antimicrobial activity of Miconia ligustroides (Melastomataceae). From the n-hexane extract of the aerial parts of M. ligustroides, the following compounds were identified by GC-MS as the main constituents: n-docosan, spinacene, n-tetratetracontane, *β-sitosterol* and *β-amyrin*. A mixture of ursolic acid and oleanoic acid was isolated from the dichloromethane extract of the aerial parts of *M. ligustroides*. These compounds were purified using HPLC and their structures were elucidated using spectroscopic data (^{1}H NMR, ^{13}C NMR, IR and MS). In addition to the crude extracts (*n-hexane*, dichloromentane and ethanol), the antimicrobial activity of the pure substances (ursolic acid, oleanolic acid and *β-sitosterol*) and semi-synthetic derivatives obtained from ursolic acid were also evaluated. The microorganisms selected for the tests were: *Bacillus cereus* (ATCC 14579), *Vibrio cholerae* (ATCC 9458), *Salmonella choleraesius* (ATCC 10708), *Klebsiella pneumoniae* (ATCC 10031), *Klebsiella pneumoniae* (ATCC 700603), *Streptococcus pneumoniae* (ATCC 6305) and the following clinical isolates: *Pseudomonas aeruginosa*, *Escherichia coli*, *Enterococcus faecalis* and *Staphylococcus aureus*. To assess the antimicrobial activity, the broth microdilution method was used to determine the minimum concentration (MIC). With regard to the extracts evaluated, the best activities were obtained against the microorganisms *B. cereus* and *S. pneumoniae*. In the evaluation of the pure substances, ursolic and oleanolic acids were active against the microorganism B. *cereus*. The substance *β-sitosterol* showed no activity against the selected microorganisms. The MIC values obtained for the derivatives obtained from ursolic acid generally showed that they did not potentiate the effects of antimicrobial activity when compared to the effects presented by ursolic acid when evaluated separately.

Keywords: *Miconia ligustroides,* antibacterial activity, ursolic acid, oleanolic acid.

CHAPTER 1

INTRODUCTION

1.1. General Aspects

Systematic research to obtain new substances for therapeutic purposes can be carried out using various processes. The most commonly used are the synthesis of new molecules, molecular modification of natural or synthetic substances with defined pharmacological properties, extraction, isolation and purification of new compounds from natural sources, especially plants, which are an inexhaustible source of potentially active substances. The use of medicinal plants for therapeutic purposes dates back to the dawn of civilisation, from the moment man awoke to consciousness and began a long journey of handling, adapting and modifying natural resources for his own benefit [1].

There are still many communities and ethnic groups today, especially those with less favoured socio-economic conditions, who use medicinal plants as their main, and often only, resource for relieving their ailments [2].

In recent years, there has been a resurgence of interest in plants as sources of new therapeutic agents. Large pharmaceutical companies have increased their research into plant extracts in order to discover new active substances [3], making natural products of plant origin an important source in the discovery of new drugs. According to literature data, 52% of the 868 drugs launched on the market during 1981-2002 have traces of or were inspired by natural products, of which 5% are of natural origin, 23% are derived from natural products, 4% are synthetic compounds derived from parts of natural product molecules and 20% are synthetic compounds modelled on known natural products (natural product analogues). In certain therapeutic areas, the use of

natural products is even higher: 78 per cent of antimicrobial compounds and 74 per cent of anticancer compounds are of natural origin or inspired by them [4].

Compounds of natural origin can play four important roles in modern pharmacology:

a) Providing useful medicines that are difficult, if not impossible, to produce and sell in synthetic form (e.g. digitalis);

b) From natural sources, basic compounds are obtained which can be slightly modified to make them more effective or less toxic (e.g. variations on the morphine molecule);

c) To serve as prototypes or models for synthetic medicines that maintain the physiological activities of the original compounds, such as procaine [5];

d) Offering a partially elaborated product of a drug that is difficult to obtain, such as stigmasterol, which is abundant in soya oil and has no therapeutic value, can be transformed by a relatively simple process into hydrocortisone or similar corticosteroids, compounds that occur in small quantities in nature [6].

The great progress made in the pharmaceutical industry in recent decades has obscured the extraordinary role medicinal plants have played, are playing and will play in therapeutics. Furthermore, the use of medicinal plants is booming in both developed and developing countries [7].

It is estimated that there are between 250,000 and 500,000 plant species on our planet [8]. In this context, ethnopharmacology acts as an extremely important tool in the study and research of new drugs of plant origin. Furthermore, the molecular diversity of the plant kingdom is still considered almost limitless, despite scientific advances [9]. It is therefore quite logical to valorise folk wisdom by providing evidence of plants with therapeutic effects as the initial stage of these research projects [10].

It is to be assumed that as research continues, hundreds of active ingredients extracted from plants will enrich the available therapeutic arsenal, as well as stimulating chemistry professionals to synthesise similar or analogous products [7]. It is known that most of the species used in developing countries have not yet been studied and so their chemical composition, pharmacological action and toxicity are unknown, representing a promising field to be explored [11].

Brazil has an immense availability of these resources, which need to be studied from a chemical and therapeutic point of view. Such studies must be carried out urgently due to the decline and imbalance that ecosystems are suffering (which leads to the consequent extinction of species). It is also important that Brazilian institutions and researchers carry out such studies in an attempt to prevent foreign laboratories from taking advantage of the lack of biodiversity regulations to obtain natural substances or derivatives used in popular and indigenous medicine, without paying anything to the country of origin. Examples can be cited, such as marapuama (Ptychopetalum olacoides), an Amazonian plant patented in Japan as a remedy for sexual impotence, or quebra-pedra (Phyllanthus nirun) patented in the USA for the treatment of hepatitis. In these cases, only the laboratories make a profit, passing on the high costs of industrialised medicines to the population, and the countries from which the original substances are taken end up losing billions of dollars in royalties [12].

1.2. **The Melastomataceae family and the genus** Miconia

The Melastomataceae is one of the most important families of Neotropical flora, with between 4,200 and 5,000 species, grouped into 11 tribes and 185 genera [13]. In Brazil, there are around 68 genera and 1,500 species, distributed from the Amazon to Rio Grande do Sul. Among the genera that occur in Brazil, Miconia stands out as the largest genus, with approximately 1000 species, distributed throughout Tropical America and especially concentrated in the Andes [14,15]. Around 250 species are represented in Brazil, 53 of which occur in the state of São Paulo [16]. No comprehensive botanical analysis has appeared since Cogniaux's family monograph in 1891 [17]. The genus shows great diversity in its trichomes, anthers and seed morphology, and can be characterised, among the others in the Miconieae tribe, by its multi-flowered, cymose terminal inflorescences, with rounded to obtuse petals at the apex [16]. According to Judd, these characteristics are all simpleiomorphic and this is why the genus has presented taxonomic problems [18]. Recent work on the genus is limited to floristic surveys [16, 19-24] or tribal positioning [14, 25]. In this way, chemical studies can be important auxiliary tools as a source of taxonomic evidence in an attempt to clarify generic and specific limits.

1.3. **Botanical data of** Miconia ligustroides (DC) Naudin

Popularly known as jacatirão-do-brejo, *Miconia ligustroides* is a shrub that varies in height from 1 to 4 metres, up to trees around 8 metres high. Its branches, petioles, inflorescence axes, hypanthium and calyx are moderately to densely covered in stellate-furfuraceous indumentum, later glabrescent to glabrous. Leaves with petiole 0.2-1 mm; blade 2.5-10x1-4 cm, chartaceous, oval, elliptic or oblong-lanceolate, base rounded, narrowly attenuate to occasionally subcordate,

obtuse to acute-acuminate apex, slightly upturned margin, suprabasal or basal acral veins; upper surface glabrous, lower surface in young leaves covered with a stellate-furfaceous indumentum,

then glabrous. Panicles 4-10 cm. Flowers pentamerous; hypanthium about 2mm; calyx deciduous, with membranaceous inner laciniae, lobed, triangular outer laciniae much reduced; petals white, pink in bud, glabrous. Stamens dimorphic, white; thecae 2.5-3 mm, ventral connective pore of the antisepal stamens dorsally thickened and sub-calcareous, antepetals basally trilobed. Ovary 3-4 locular, glabrous; stipe slightly thickened at apex. Berries atropurpous, about 04 seeds per loculus [16].

Distribution and habitat**:** It occurs from Ceará to Santa Catarina. In São Paulo it is found in savannahs, on the edge of forests and in marshy places [16].

Miconia ligustroides (Table 1 and Figure 1) is a polymorphic species, varying mainly in the shape and size of the leaves and the presence or absence of indumentum on the adult parts of the plant. It has similarities with M. *minutiflora* (Bonpl.) DC. from which it differs mainly because the latter has generally larger leaves with a greater number of veins, antepetal stamen connective with a more pronounced and acute calcar, petals with glandular trichomes, and calyx with ciliated internal laciniae. Various materials belonging to this species, including some cited by Hoehne (1922) - Frazão s.n. (SP 10799) and Navarro de Andrade s.n. (SP 10821) - were identified as *M. candolleana triana, a* synonym of *M. cinnamomifolia* [16].

Table 1. Characteristics of *Miconia ligustroides (DC.) Naudin*

Family	**Melastomataceae**
Size	Tree
Environment	Cerrado, cerradão, riparian forest
Flowering time	September
Fruiting season	March

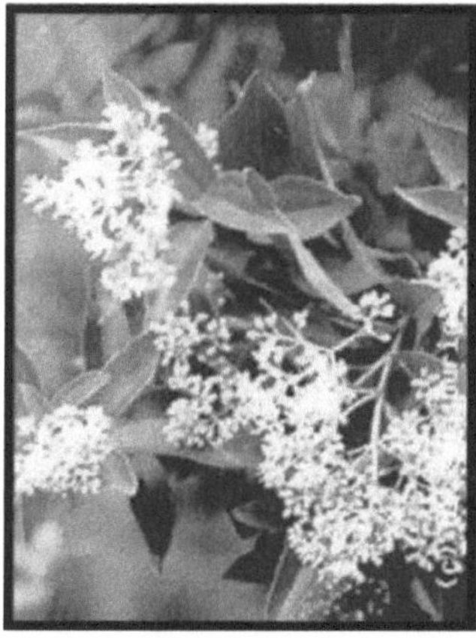

Figure 1: Miconia ligustroides (Melastomataceae)
Source: Flora do Cerrado do Estado de São Paulo [16].

1.4. Ursolic and oleanolic acid - substances with biological potential

Ursolic acid (UA) and its isomer oleanolic acid (OA) (Figure 2) are triterpene compounds widely found in plants used in human food and medicinal herbs, in the form of free or aglyconated acid or as triterpenoid saponins [26-29]. According to Price et al. [26] saponins can be chemically as an aglycone attached to one or more sugar chains. There are two groups of saponins, one containing a steroid aglycone and the other containing a triterpenoid aglycone. Like steroids, triterpenoids have various biological effects.

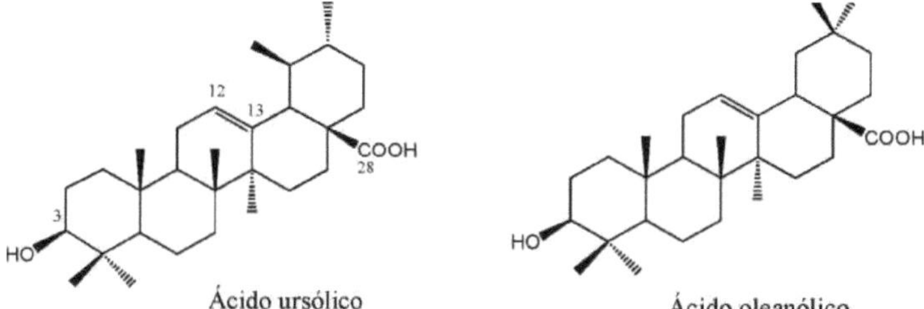

Figure 2: Chemical structures of ursolic and oleanolic acids

Numerous biological activities related to UA and AO have been studied from extracts taken from various popular or medicinal plants, including hepatoprotective, anti-inflammatory, anti-ulcer, antimicrobial, hypoglycaemic, anti-malarial and anti-tumour [27-33]. These triterpenoids have hepatoprotective properties by reducing necrosis of liver parenchymal cells, steatosis, fibrosis, preventing chronic cirrhosis and intensifying liver regeneration [30,34,35]. A reduction in the effects of carbon tetrachloride (CCI4) on the liver of rats has also been observed through oral administration of OA [36] and through nanosuspensions containing OA [37]. Since the 1960s, the anti-inflammatory and inhibitory effects of UA and OA on rat paw oedema caused by carrageenan and arthritis have been reported [31,32,38-41]. The mechanisms involved in their anti-inflammatory effects have been attributed to the inhibition of histamine [42,43], the inhibition of lipoxygenase and cyclooxygenase activity [44,45], the inhibition of elastase [46], reducing some inflammatory factors produced during the aricidonic acid cascade [42,47].

Both AU and AO, as well as their derivatives, have been shown to be efficient anti-ulcer and analgesic agents [32,34,48,49].

The AU and AO present in Symphonia globulifera seeds have demonstrated antimicrobial activities [50], inhibiting the growth of Staphylococcus aureus, gram-negative bacteria and Microsporium lenosum [34]. AU also reduces the cytopathic effects of cells exposed to the Herpes simplex virus [51]. AO-type saponins have also exhibited a broad spectrum of antifungal activity, especially against Candida glabrata [33].

Treatment with AO lowers the blood glucose level of alloxan-induced diabetic mice. The rise in blood glucose caused by adrenaline or glucose was also attenuated by treatment with AU and with AO [32].

The hypolipidaemic and anti-atherosclerosis activities of UA and OA have also been described, giving rise to considerable clinical interest [34, 52, 53].

Antiparasitic activities have been found against Plasmodium falciparum species [54], Trypanosoma sp [74,55] and Leishmania species [56]. AU has been identified as one of the active components against dental caries in vitro [34]; effects on periodontal pathogens [57], antitubercular potential against Mycobactrium tuberculosis [58], antiviral against HIV [32] and antifertility [59].

Both AU and AO are considered relatively non-toxic when used in various experimental models [34, 41,65].

Research indicates that AU is a potent inhibitor of DNA polymerase alpha in cattle, DNA polymerase beta in mice and human DNA Topoisomerases I and II. AU has also shown a moderate inhibitory effect on plant DNA polymerase II and Human Immunodeficiency Virus reverse transcriptase [61,62]. According to Ovesna et al [32], AU and AO can act at various stages in tumour development: such as inhibiting tumourigenesis, inhibiting tumour promotion and inducing tumour cell differentiation. They effectively inhibit angiogenesis, tumour cell invasion and metastasis. They are able to induce apoptosis in tumour cells and prevent the malignant transformation of normal cells [28]. In short, AU and AO have the potential to be used as adjuvants in cancer therapy [63,64].

The mechanisms by which AU and AO suppress tumour promotion are not known, but may occur due to the inhibition of inflammation produced by tumour promoters [65]; the suppression of oncogenic expression [34]; the induction of differentiation [66] and modulation of the body's defence system, such as antioxidant potential and immune functions [67].

The mechanisms involved in the antitumour activity of AU and AO may also be related to their ability to inhibit DNA replication, tyrosine kinase activity [28], inducible nitric oxide synthesis [68], matrix metalloproteinase-9 [69] and the expression of lipoxygenase [70] and cyclooxygenase-2. On the other hand, AU and AO induce morphological changes and internucleosomal DNA fragmentation, characteristic of apoptotic cell death, which is mediated by the activation of caspases [71] and the release of intracellular $Ca+^{2}$ [72] and cytochrome C [67,71].

There is great therapeutic interest in UA and AO due to their chemopreventive properties [63]. The use of triterpenoid compounds has been recommended for skin cancer therapy in Japan [73], and the preparation

Pharmaceuticals containing AU and AO are authorised for the treatment of non-lymphatic leukaemia [34]. However, more studies are needed to better understand the molecular mechanisms involved in their chemopreventive effects so that they can be used safely and effectively.

1.5 General considerations about the microorganisms studied

The growing emergence of multiresistant pathogenic microorganisms responsible for many deaths, especially hospital-acquired infections, has prompted the search for new drugs. The entry and multiplication of a microorganism in the body, causing damage to the host, characterises an infection. When this organism is able to circumvent the host's normal defences in order to install the infection, we say that it is a pathogen.

Infections can be opportunistic, when human defences are weakened, allowing the entry of organisms that would not normally cause harm to a healthy individual, or hospital-acquired infections known as nosocomial.

Antimicrobials are chemical substances that inhibit the growth of or destroy microorganisms. They can be produced from other microorganisms, such as atypical bacteria and fungi, or synthesised in whole or in part. Currently, antibiotics are among the most widely used drugs in outpatient therapy and in hospitals.

The indiscriminate use of these drugs has led to the development of bacterial resistance and, consequently, the emergence of superinfections by multiresistant germs [76,77]

Below are some of the characteristics of the pathogens used in this research.

Pseudomonas aeruginosa [77,78]

P. aeruginosa is a typically opportunistic germ that can cause various diseases. Localised infections caused by this microorganism as a result of surgery or burns can result in severe bacteraemia, and urinary infections associated with the use of catheters are common. Most cystic fibrosis patients are colonised by P. aeruginosa, although they rarely suffer bacteraemia. It is assumed that this resistance is due to the presence of high levels of serum antibodies. In some of these patients, the bacterium causes fatal pneumonia. Severe pneumonia can also occur in patients who use contaminated respirators. P. *aeruginosa* can cause keratitis as a result of eye surgery. Although rare, it can cause meningitis after lumbar punctures and endocarditis after heart surgery.

Several studies have shown that *P. aeruginosa* usually colonises the respiratory tract after some illnesses or the use of catheters. This seems to occur because the epithelial cell loses fibronectin, a protein that blocks the bacteria from adhering to the normal epithelium. Adherence is mediated by fimbriae or perhaps by the bacterium's glycocalyx.

P. aeruginosa produces a series of substances that could be involved in the pathogenesis of infection. Toxin A is the most toxic, and its mechanism of action is identical to that of diphtheria toxin, i.e. it blocks protein synthesis by inhibiting the elongation factor EF-2. Samples that don't produce toxin A are less virulent. This bacterium is resistant to the bactericidal power of serum, but is very sensitive to phagocytosis in the presence of opsonins.

P. aeruginosa is naturally resistant to various beta- lactam antibiotics, as well as tetracyclines, chloramphenicol, cotrimoxazole and others. The most effective antibiotics are gentamicin, amikacin, some semi-synthetic penicillins (carbenicillin) and polymyxin. The bacteria can acquire resistance to any of these therapeutic agents (with the exception of polymyxin) through mutations or the acquisition of resistance plasmids. An antibiogram is recommended for selecting the antibiotic to be used in treatment.

Klebsiela pneumoniae [77,79]

K. pneumoniae is normally found in the intestines. It is one of the few Gram-negative bacilli to cause lobar pneumonia. Alcoholics are particularly susceptible to infection. Pneumonia is usually localised in the upper lobes, accompanied by necrosis which can lead to cavity formation. Not infrequently, the bacterium is also found in association with urinary tract infections, endocarditis and various types of post-surgical infections. Some statistics show that K. pneumoniae may be responsible for 10 per cent of hospital-acquired infections. The hospital sample is often resistant to most antimicrobials. More than 95 per cent of Klebsiella samples isolated from different clinical specimens are K. pneumoniae.

Streptococcus pneumoniae [80,81]

The main diseases caused by S. pneumoniae are acute pneumonia, otitis media, sinusitis, bacterial meningitis and endocarditis. Around 90 per cent of bacterial pneumonia is caused by S. pneumoniae. Normally the pneumococcus sample responsible for pneumonia is found in the patient's upper airways, from where it is aspirated into the pulmonary alveoli. Once in the alveoli, the bacterium proliferates and causes the inflammatory reaction characteristic of penumonia. The pleura can be affected, resulting in (sterile) pleural effusion or, more rarely, empyema. Obviously, infection only occurs if the pneumococcus is able to escape phagocytosis. In untreated patients who survive the infection, pneumonia follows a typical course that ends in a spontaneous cure a week after its onset. The cure coincides with the appearance of specific serum opsonins that promote phagocytosis of the germ involved in the process. Approximately 30% of patients with pneumonia have bacteraemia, and pneumococcus can be isolated by

easily from the blood. In some cases, pneumonia can have complications such as arthritis, endocarditis and meningitis.

Normal people are very resistant to pneumococcal lung infection due to their efficient defence mechanisms. These include the epiglottal reflex, ciliary movement, cough reflex, lymphatic drainage and the macrophages that patrol the alveoli. Thus, an individual usually acquires pneumonia when the mechanisms that protect them are compromised, which can happen as a result of viral infections of the upper airways, alcohol intoxication, congestive heart failure and other factors.

Pneumococcal otitis and sinusitis are usually secondary to functional alterations of the middle ear and sinuses and are caused by pneumococci normally present in the upper airways. Meningitis, as well as arising from bacterial pneumonia, can be a complication of otitis, sinusitis and endocarditis. The pneumococcus' sensitivity to antibiotics, as well as its ability to acquire resistance, are very similar to those of S. pyogenes. The antibiotic of choice is still penicillin G. Although tetracycline and chloramphenicol are active, the isolation of samples resistant to these drugs is now quite common. It should also be noted that in some countries (Australia and South Africa) penicillin-resistant pneumococcal samples have emerged, as well as those with multiple resistance. The resistance of these samples to penicillin is not due to the production of penicillase.

Staphylococcus aureus [82,83]

S. aureus causes disease through the production of toxins or direct invasion and destruction of tissue. The clinical manifestations of some staphylococcal diseases result almost exclusively from toxin activity, while other diseases result from the proliferation of the microorganism, leading to abscess formation and tissue destruction (e.g. skin infection, endocarditis, pneumonia, empyema, osteomyelitis and septic arthritis). In the presence of foreign bodies (e.g. pins, catheters, shunts, prosthetic valves or joints), significantly fewer staphylococci are needed to establish disease. Similarly, patients with congenital diseases associated with an impaired chemotherapeutic or phagocytic response (e.g. Job-Buckley syndrome, Wiskott-Aldrich syndrome and chronic granulomatous disease) are more susceptible to staphylococcal diseases.

The antibiotic of choice is oxacillin, or vancomycin for oxacillin-resistant strains.

Bacillus cereus [84,85]

Bacillus species other than B. anthracis are mainly opportunistic pathogens with little capacity for virulence. Although many of these species have been found to cause disease, B. cereus is clearly the most important pathogen, causing gastroenteritis, eye infections and sepsis related to intravenous catheters.

Because gastroenteritis caused by B. cereus is short and uncomplicated, only symptomatic treatment is sufficient. Vancomycin, clindamycin, ciprofloxacin and gentamicin can be used to treat infections. Rapid consumption of food after cooking and appropriate refrigeration of what has not been consumed can prevent food-borne infection.

Vibrio cholerae [86,87]

Infection caused by V. cholerae can range from asymptomatic

colonisation, or mild diarrhoea, to rapidly fatal severe diarrhoea. The clinical manifestations of cholera begin on average two to three days after ingesting the bacteria, with the abrupt onset of watery diarrhoea and vomiting. As more fluid is lost, the stool specimens become colourless and odourless, free of protein and flecked with mucus ("rice water" stools). Severe loss of fluids and electrolytes can lead to dehydration, metabolic acidosis (loss of bicarbonate) and hypokalaemia and hypovolaemic shock (loss of potassium) with cardiac arrhythmia and kidney failure. The mortality rate is 60 per cent in untreated patients and less than 1 per cent in patients promptly treated with replacement of fluid and electrolyte loss. Cholera can heal spontaneously after a few days of symptoms. Gastroenteritis caused by other serotypes of V. cholerae is mild and is not associated with epidemics. Fluid and electrolyte replacement is crucial. Antibiotics reduce the bacterial load and exotoxin production, as well as the duration of diarrhoea. Doxycycline (adults), trimethoprim sulphamethoxazole (children) or furazolidine (pregnant women) are administered.

Enerococcus [82,88,89]

Enterococcus is an important cause of nosocomial infections associated with urinary tract infections, endocarditis, intra-abdominal and pelvic infections, as well as catheter infections, surgical process infections and central nervous system infections. The most common species of Enterococcus are faecalis and faecium. Both are capable of producing biofilms, which consist of a population of cells that irreversibly attack various living or non-living surfaces in a hydrated matrix of exopolymeric substances. Many genetic and environmental factors are associated or have been proposed to be associated with biofilm production. E. faecalis is a Gram-positive bacterium, a member of the lactic acid bacteria group, and oxidative stress is one of the main challenges the bacterium faces during the infectious process. Since the first use of antimicrobials to hinder bacterial resistance, it has progressively increased and has accelerated over the last 10 years. Antibiotic-resistant genes have been present at low levels prior to the introduction of antibiotics and largely by increasing the selectivity of antibiotic use. Bacterial exposure, not only in humans, but also in food, animals and the environment, has been on the rise. The increasing mobility of people, food and animals is another factor. Examples of this are the international epidemic of CTX-M extended-spectrum beta-lactamase genotypes. The response given to society to reduce bacterial resistance involves the prospect of reduced antibiotic use, improved infection control and the introduction of new antimicrobial agents. Although efforts are being made in all areas, there is an urgent need to increase the efficiency of interventions for some bacterial infections.

Escherichia coli [90]

A large number of E. coli are present in the gastrointestinal tract, and these bacteria are common causes of sepsis, neonatal meningitis, urinary tract infections and gastroenteritis. For example, E. coli is a Gram-negative rod most commonly isolated in patients with sepsis and is responsible for causing more than 80 per cent of all community-acquired UTIs, as well as many hospital-acquired infections and an important cause of gastroenteritis in developing countries. Most infections (except neonatal meningitis and gastroenteritis) are endogenous: that is, organisms that are part of the normal microbiota are able to establish an infection when the patient's defences are compromised. Enteric pathogens are treated symptomatically unless disseminated disease occurs. Antibiotic therapy is guided by in vitro susceptibility tests. Appropriate infection control practices are used to reduce the risk of nosocomial infections (e.g. restricting the use of urinary catheters). Maintain high hygiene conditions to reduce the risk of exposure to strains that cause gastroenteritis and cook food properly to reduce the risk of EHEC infections.

Salmonella Choleraesuis [91,92,93,94]

It is estimated that 1.3 million people a year contract illnesses caused by Salmonella in the United States, leading to the deaths of 500 people a year [92]. Most infections caused by Salmonella species are acquired by eating contaminated food (poultry, eggs, some types of meat and dairy products are the most common sources of infection) [91]. In recent years, S. choleraesuis has been frequently isolated from pig meat [91]. The main complication is the development of an aneurysm that can lead to death [93]. In recent years, the greatest aggravation is the resistance of this type of Salmonella to some antibiotics [93, 94]. Most infections caused by Salmonella can be controlled by the proper preparation of poultry and eggs (fully cooked) and by avoiding the contamination of other foods with raw poultry products.

CHAPTER 2

BIBLIOGRAPHICAL REVIEW OF THE GENUS Miconia

From a chemical-pharmacological point of view, few studies have been carried out on species of the genus Miconia. In chemical studies, the isolation of quinones, coumarins and triterpenes predominates [101-103]. The studies carried out on Miconia species are listed in Table 2. Biological activity studies carried out in our laboratories with Miconia species and isolated substances have led to promising results (Table 3).

Table 2. Miconia species that have undergone some kind of biological test.

Species	Extract and substances active	Type of biological activity	References
M. *attenuatus*	Ellagic acid	Antifungal	95 a 99
M. ciliata	Ethanolic extract of leaves	Sedative activity	100
M. eriodonta	Primin/Miconidin	Antimicrobial/Antitumour/ Trypanocidal	101 e 102
M. laevigata	Ellagic acid	Antifungal	95 a 99
M. lepidota	Benzoquinones	Cytotoxic/Antitumour	103
M. macrothyrsa	Ellagic acid	Antifungal	95 a 99
M. macroti	Ellagic acid	Antifungal	95 a 99
M. myriantha	Branches/leaves	Antifungal	99
M. prasina	Ellagic acid	Antifungal	95 a 00
M. pulgeriana	Arjunolic acid	Antifungal	114
M. racenosa	Methanolic extract of wood	Anti-malarial activity	104
M. tamonea	Ellagic acid	Antifungal	95 a 99
M. cabucu	Ethanolic and dichloromethane extracts	Antimicrobial	115

Table 3. Species of Miconia that have undergone biological tests in our laboratories.

Species	Extract and active substances	Biological activity Rated	References
M. albicans	Hexane, dichloromethane and ethanolic extracts of the aerial parts	Analgesic	105
M. *albicans*	Ursolic acid and oleanoic acid	Analgesic	106
M. fallax	Dichloromethane extract of the aerial parts	Trypanocidal	74
M. fallax	Ethanolic extract of the aerial parts	Analgesic	107
M. fallax	Ethanolic extract	Antitumour	108
M. fallax	Ursolic acid and Oleanolic acid	Antimutagenic	109

M. ligustroides	Hexanic, dichloromethanic and ethanolic extracts of the aerial parts	Analgesic	110
M. ligustroides *M. sellowiana*	Ursolic acid and Oleanolic acid	Trypanocidal	102
M. rubiginosa	Hexane, dichloromethane and ethanolic extracts of the aerial parts	Analgesic	111
M. sellowiana *M. albicans* *M. stenostachia*	Ursolic acid and Oleanolic acid and Derivatives	Antimicrobial	112
M. stenostachya	Dichloromethane extract of the aerial parts	Trypanocidal	74
M. stenostachya *M. rubiginosa* *M. fallax* *M. albicans*	Hexane, dichloromethane and ethanolic extracts of the aerial parts	Antifungal	108
M. stenostachya *M. rubiginosa* *M. fallax* *M. albicans*	Hexanolic, dichloromethanic and ethanolic extracts of the aerial parts	Antimicrobial	113

CHAPTER 3

OBJECTIVES

The objectives of this study were:

a) Obtaining the crude extracts in n-hexane, dichloromethane and ethanol of the plant species Miconia ligustroides belonging to the Melastomataceae family;
b) Obtaining the pure substances ursolic acid and oleanoic acid, present in the dichloromentane extract of M. ligustroides;
c) Evaluation of the antimicrobial activity of crude extracts and pure substances;
d) Obtaining semi-synthetic derivatives of ursolic acid with a view to optimising antimicrobial activity evaluation results.

CHAPTER 4

MATERIALS AND METHODS

4.1 Instrument specifications

- The NMR spectra were recorded on a Bruker DPX and XRD spectrometer operating at 400 MHz for ^{1}H and 100 MHz for ^{13}C.

- The HPLC was carried out on a Shimadzu LC-6A chromatograph with UV-visible detector model SPD-6A, with SCL6B integrator C- R6A controller;

- The samples were concentrated in a rotary evaporator under reduced pressure (Marconi, MA 120).

- CCDC developer: UV lamp (254 and 366nm), Mineralight, model UVGL-25.

- The GC-MS analyses were carried out on a shimadzu QP 2010 chromatograph, DB-17 MS column (30m x 0.25mm x 0.25μ) *and* comparison with data from the library

- Mass spectra were obtained on an ultrOTOFq mass spectrometer (Bruker Daltonics, Billerica, MA, USA) equipped with an electrospray ionisation (ESI) source. Analyses were carried out in the negative analysis mode by directly infusing solutions of the sample in MeOH: H_2O 8:2.

4.2 Specifications of chromatographic columns and stationary phases

- Fractionation by liquid vacuum column (LVC) was carried out on a glass column (h12 cm x d20 cm) equipped with a vacuum outlet at its lower end. A mixture of celite + active charcoal in the ratio (3:1 m/m) was used as the stationary phase to purify the UA.

- Glass plates (5 x 20 and 10 x 20 cm) coated with Merck silica gel 60 GF_{254} were used to prepare the comparative thin layer chromatography (CCDC) plates.

of suspension in water at a ratio of 1:2 (m/v) with a Desaga spreader, forming a 0.25

mm thick layer of silica. These plates were then activated in an oven at 100 °C before being used.

- A 5μm silica SHIMADZU column was used for the HPLC (20 x 250 mm mobile phase: hexane: isopropyl alcohol (98:2 v/v), flow 9 mL/min, UV detector: 225 nm). These conditions were used to purify ursolic and oleanolic acids.

- The GC-MS analyses were carried out on a Shimadzu QP 2010 apparatus, DB-17 MS column (30m x 0.25mm x 0.25μ), injection temperature 260°C, He carrier gas (1.40 ml/min), column temperature - ramp 120°C to 260C (0-5 min - 20"C/min), 260"C to 280"C (5-9 min - 2'C/min), 280C to 290C (9-20 min).

3.1 Solvent and reagent specifications

- The solvents used were of P.A. and CLAE purity.

- Aldrich deuterated solvents were used to obtain the IH and ^{13}C NMR spectra.

- To reveal the chromatographic plates, the developer was used: sulphuric acid (8:2 solution in distilled water). Nebulisation with sulphuric acid was followed by heating on a plate (Marconi, MA 239) at 100°C until the spots corresponding to the substances present appeared.

3.2 . Experimental Part

3.2.1 Collection and identification of plant material

The aerial parts of M. ligustroides were collected by Prof. Dr. Wilson Roberto Cunha in October 2005, in the Serra de

Canoas, on the border between the states of São Paulo and Minas Gerais, NE sector, near the Tancredo Neves Highway [Franca (SP) - Claraval (MG)]. The botanical identification of the species was carried out by Prof. Dr Ângela Borges Martins. Dr Ângela Borges Martins from the Botany Institute at UNICAMP. An exsiccate of the plant material (UEC 10821) is deposited in the ICB herbarium (UNICAMP).

3.2.2 Obtaining crude extracts of M. ligustroides

The aerial parts of the plant were dried and stabilised in a circulating air oven (40°C) and ground to a powder in a knife mill. The resulting M. ligustroides powder (0.5kg) was extracted three times over seven days at room temperature by maceration with the solvents n-hexane, dichloromethane and then ethanol. These extracts were evaluated for their antimicrobial activity. The masses of the crude extracts obtained are shown in Table 4.

Table 4: Masses of the crude extracts obtained from M. ligustroides.

Species	Extract	Mass (g)	Income
M. *ligustroides*	n-hexane	4,3	0,86%
	Dichloromethane	6,5	1,3%
	Ethanolic	8,6	1,72%

3.2.3 Analysis of the crude extracts of M. ligustroides

3.2.3.1 Study of the n-hexane extract of M. ligustroides

A sample of the n-hexane extract (1.0 g) was filtered through a column containing celite + active carbon and eluted with dichloromethane, which was then evaporated in a rotaevaporator. The resulting fraction (200 mg) was then analysed using GC-MS to identify the main constituents.

4.4.3.2 Isolation of ursolic and oleanoic acid from the extract in dichloromethane

This extract (6.0 g) was subjected to filter column chromatography (CLV), using a mixture of celite + active carbon (3:1 w/w) as the stationary phase and dichloromethane as the mobile phase. The aim of this procedure was to purify ursolic and oleanolic acid for subsequent biological tests and semi-synthesis reactions. 5 litres of dichloromethane were used as the mobile phase, which after rotaevaporation provided 0.5g of amorphous solid material. This material was recrystallised in n-hexane/ethyl acetate and subsequently coded as ML-1. As it was a mixture, part of this material was submitted to CLAE in order to isolate its components.

4.4.4 . Obtaining ursolic acid derivatives

4.4.4.1. Ursolic acid esterification reaction

Ursolic acid (20 mg) was esterified with diazomethane according to the usual methodology [99], using N-methyl-N-nitroso-p-toluene-sulfonamide (Diazald) as the starting material for the synthesis of diazomethane. The reaction was carried out with the aim of obtaining a derivative for biological testing **(Scheme 1).**

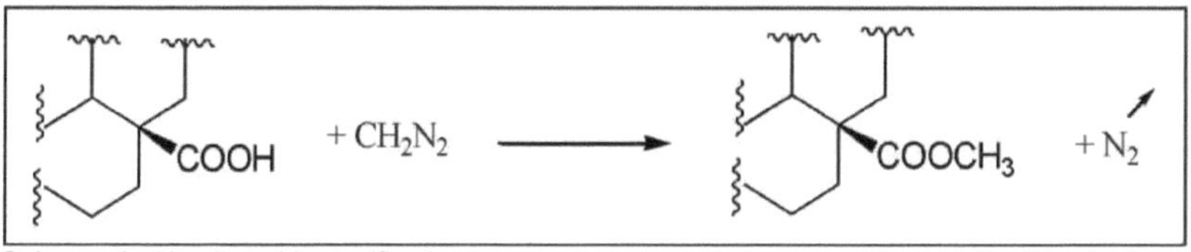

COOH $+ CH_2N_2$ → $COOCH_3$ $+ N_2$

Scheme 1 - Ursolic acid esterification reaction

3.2.3.2 Acetylation reaction of ursolic acid

Ursolic acid (50 mg) was acetylated using acetic anhydride (2.0 mL) and pyridine (0.5 mL) to obtain a derivative for biological testing. The mixture was refluxed at 70°C for 1 hour, then toluene (10 mL) was added to the reaction mixture and it was rotaevaporated, the process being repeated 5 times to remove the pyridine. Afterwards, dichloromethane (10 mL) was added and the reaction medium was rotaevaporated, the process being repeated 5 times in order to eliminate the toluene **(Scheme 2).**

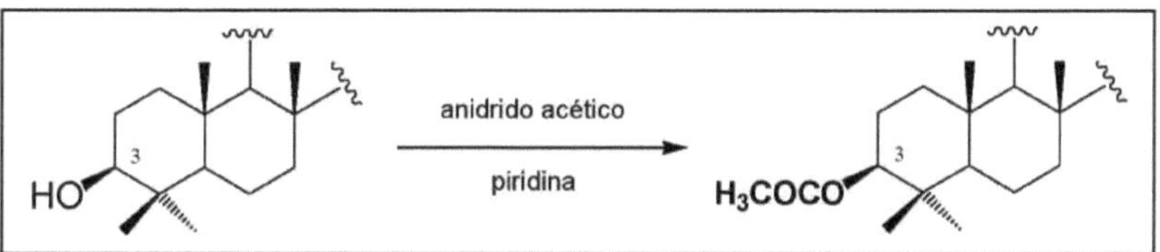

Scheme 2 - Acetylation reaction of ursolic acid

4.4.4.3. Reaction to obtain the salt derived from ursolic acid

In order to obtain derivatives for evaluation in antimicrobial activity tests, the potassium salt of ursolic acid was prepared (Scheme 3). ursolic acid (50 mg) was treated with a 2% solution of KOH in acetone/water (1:1) at room temperature for 30 minutes. After removing the acetone by evaporation, the resulting aqueous solution was chromatographed on a Sephadex LH-20 column. Elution was carried out with methanol, making it possible to obtain the derivative salt (30 mg) and the diagram is shown below [116].

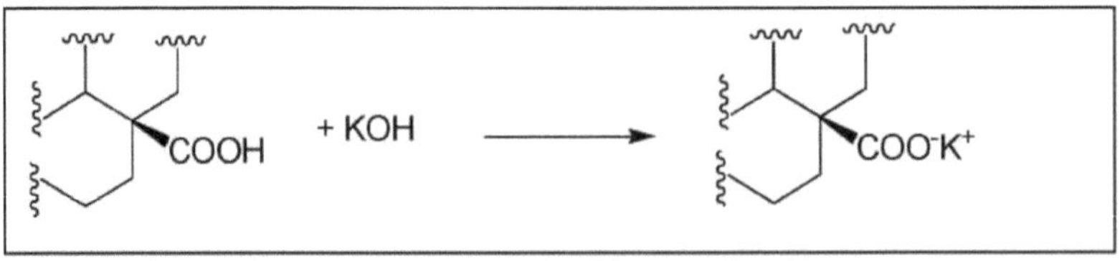

$COOH + KOH \longrightarrow COO^-K^+$

Scheme 3 - Reaction to obtain the salt derived from ursolic acid

4.4.5 . Evaluation of the antimicrobial activity of the crude extracts, isolated substances, derivatives and mixtures.

The antimicrobial activity of the crude extracts of the Miconia ligustroides species was determined using the broth microdilution method to determine the minimum inhibitory concentration (MIC) and the samples evaluated are listed in Table 5.

Table 5 - Description of the samples of crude extracts, pure substances, mixtures and semi-synthetic derivatives evaluated in the antimicrobial assays used for testing antimicrobial activity.

SAMPLES	FORM USED	EVALUATION OF ANTIMICROBIAL ACTIVITY
M. *ligustroides*	Ethanolic extract	CIM
M. ligustroides	Dichloromethane extract	CIM
M. ligustroides	Hexanic extract	CIM
Oleanolic acid	Pure Sustance (isolated from *M. ligustroides*)	CIM
Ursolic *Acid* + Ac. Oleanolic	Mixing (isolated from *M. ligustroides*)	CIM
Derived salt	Derived from ursolic acid	CIM
Ester derivative	Derived from ac. Ursolic acid	CIM
Acetate derivative	Derived from ursolic acid	CIM

4.4.5.1 Microorganisms used in the tests

The following standard strains from the American Type Culture Collection (ATCC) were used to determine the antimicrobial activity of the crude extracts, isolated substances and semi-synthetic derivatives: Bacillus cereus (ATCC 14579), Vibrio cholerae (ATCC 9458), Salmonella choleraesius (ATCC 10708), Klebsiella pneumoniae (ATCC 10031), Klebsiella pneumoniae (ATCC 700603), Streptococcus pneumoniae (ATCC 6305) and the following clinical isolates: Pseudomonas aeruginosa, Escherichia coli, Enterococcus faecalis and Staphylococcus aureus. Most of the microorganisms were kept frozen at -20°C in tryptone soya broth (TSB) containing 15% glycerol at 80%. For more demanding microorganisms, such as Streptococcus pneumoniae, sterile defibrillated sheep's blood was added to the TSB broth in equal proportions.

Table 1 - Microorganisms, origin, morphotypes and culture media used to assess antimicrobial activity.

Microorganism/Standard Strains ATCC and isolates	**Morphotype**	**Culture medium** Inoculum
Bacillus cereus ATCC 14579	Bacillus Gram-positive	Brain Heart Infusion (BHI) broth
Vibrio cholerae ATCC 9458	Bacillus Gram-negative	Brain Heart Infusion (BHI) broth
Salmonella choleraesius ATCC 10708	Bacillus Gram-negative	Brain Heart Infusion (BHI) broth
Klebsiella pneumoniae ATCC 10031	Bacillus Gram-negative	Brain Heart Infusion (BHI) broth
Klebsiella pneumoniae ATCC 700603	Bacillus Gram-negative	Brain Heart Infusion (BHI) broth
Streptococcus pneumoniae ATCC 6305	Coconut Gram-positive	Brain Heart Infusion (BHI) broth
Pseudomonas aeruginosa Clinical isolate	Bacillus Gram-negative	Brain Heart Infusion (BHI) broth
Escherichia coli Clinical isolate	Bacillus Gram-negative	Brain Heart Infusion (BHI) broth
Enterococcus faecalis Clinical isolate	Coconut Gram-positive	Brain Heart Infusion (BHI) broth
Staphylococcus aureus Clinical isolate	Coconut Gram-positive	Brain Heart Infusion (BHI) broth

4.4.5.2 Microdilution method for determining the minimum inhibitory concentration

4.4.5.2.1 Sample preparation

Solutions of the crude extracts, semi-synthetic derivatives and pure substances containing 1.0 mg/125pL in DMSO were prepared. After the substances had been completely solubilised, 1875 pL of the BHI broth described in flowchart 1 was added.

4.4.5.1.1 Preparation of the inoculum

Using a sterilised platinum loop, 24-hour cultures of the microorganisms grown in their respective culture media were transferred to tubes containing 5 mL of sterilised saline solution. These suspensions were standardised against the 0.5 tube of the McFarland scale (0.1 mL of 1.0% barium chloride + 9.9 mL of 1.0% sulphuric acid) by checking the absorbance at 625 nm and transmittance at 81 nm. Dilution was then carried out in BHI broth in order to provide the inoculum of 5 x 10^5 CFU/mL described in flowchart 1 [117].

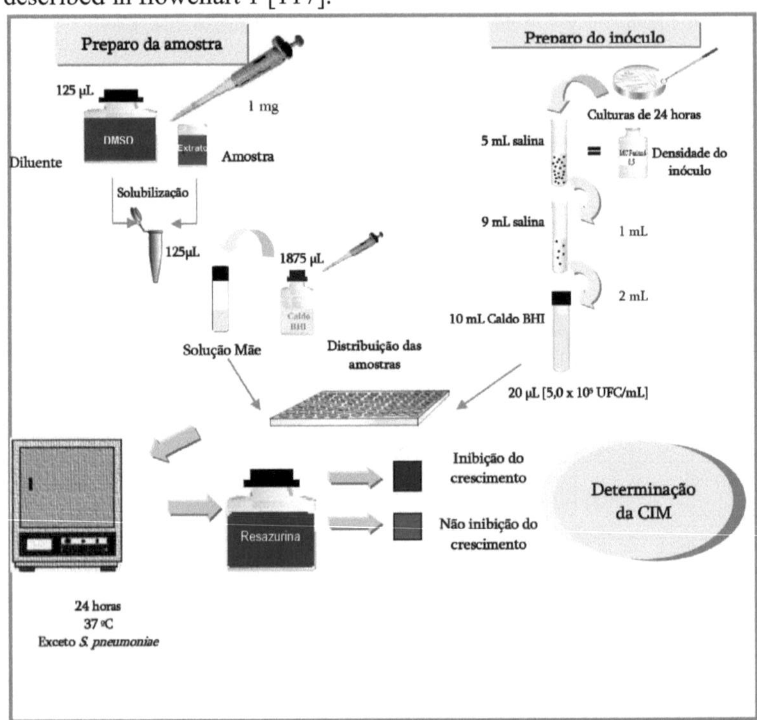

Flowchart 1 - Schematisation of sample and inoculum preparation for the Minimum Inhibitory Concentration (MIC) test

4.4.5.1.2 Preparation of positive controls

The following drugs were used as positive controls: Gentamicin for Gram-negative microorganisms, Vancomycin for Gram-positive and Imipenem for Gram-negative bacteria Klebsiella pneumoniae, Escherichia coli and Pseudomonas aeruginosa [101].

For the positive controls, the concentrations of the drugs evaluated ranged from 0.0115 μg/mL to 5.9 μg/mL.

Firstly, the antibiotic solutions were prepared at a concentration of 10 mg/mL, taking into account the potency of each antibiotic tested. Then 10 μL of this solution was transferred to a test tube containing 4,990 μL of BHI broth to obtain a concentration of 0.02 mg/mL of the solution for use.

4.4.5.1.3 Determining the antimicrobial activity of the samples

A total of 100 μL of the mixture of BHI broth, solutions of the extracts, fractions or pure substances and suspensions of the microorganisms were deposited in sterile 96-hole microplates. The samples were evaluated at the following concentrations from 10 to 1000 μg/mL. Minimum inhibitory concentrations were determined using the microplate microdilution method.

In one of the holes in each plate, the culture was checked for bacterial growth due to the absence of the antimicrobial agent. Another hole was used to check the sterility of the BHI broth and another to check the solvent used to solubilise the extracts and pure isolated substances.

The microplates were sealed with parafilm and incubated at 37°C for 24 hours. The Streptococcus pneumoniae microorganism was incubated at 37°C for 24 hours in microaerophilia. After the incubation time, 15μL of 0.01% aqueous resazurin solution was added to each hole[128]. This developer system allows immediate observation, in which the presence of a blue colour represents the absence of growth, while a red colour is interpreted as the presence of bacterial growth [118].

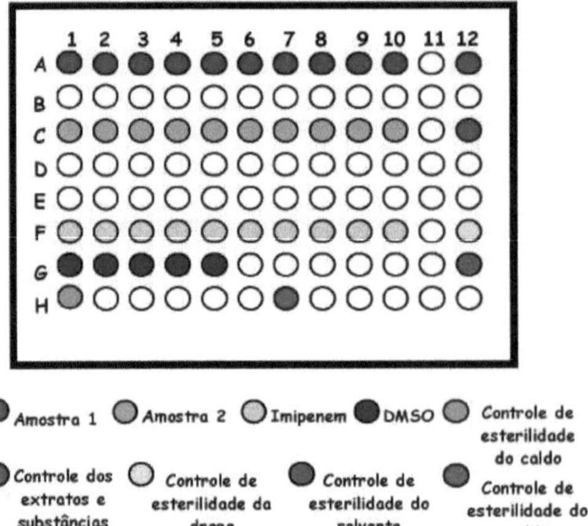

Diagram 4 - Diagram for the broth microdilution technique used to determine the MIC, according to the CLSI methodology, in a 96-hole microplate.

CHAPTER 5

RESULTS AND DISCUSSION

5.1. Analysis of the n-hexane extract of M. ligustroides by GC-MS

Using GC-MS (appendix 1), it was possible to verify the presence of esters, alcohols and long-chain hydrocarbons in the n-hexane extract of M. ligustroides. By selecting only the peaks with an area percentage above 5%, the following substances can be established as the majority constitution of the extract: n-docosane (**I**) (Tr= 11.478 min.; 34.74%; IS= 95, appendix 2), spinacene (**II**) (Tr=12.628 min.6.23%; IS=96, Annex 3), n- tetratetracontane (**III**) (Tr= 14.516 min; 18.76%; IS=97, Annex 4), β-sitosterol (**IV**) (Tr=27.292 min; 6.64%; IS=94, Annex 5) and β-amyrin (**V**) (Tr=33.319 min; 10.90%; IS=87, Annex 6).

$CH_3(CH_2)_{20}CH_3$
I

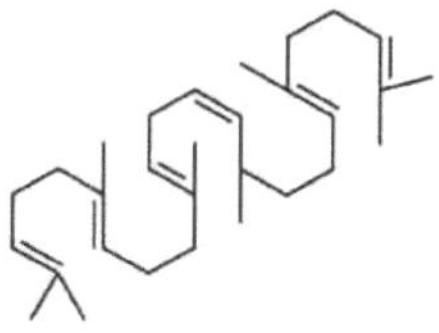

II

$CH_3(CH_2)_{42}CH_3$
III

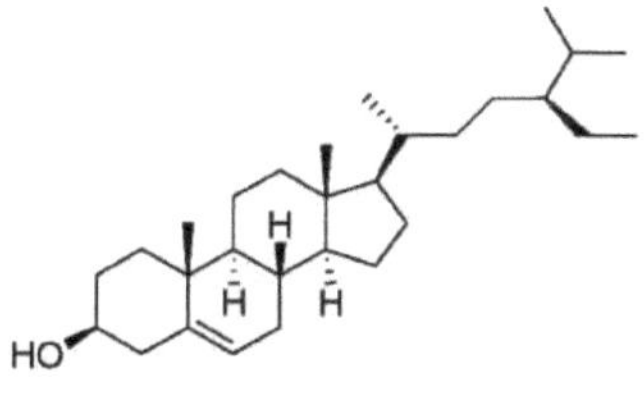

IV

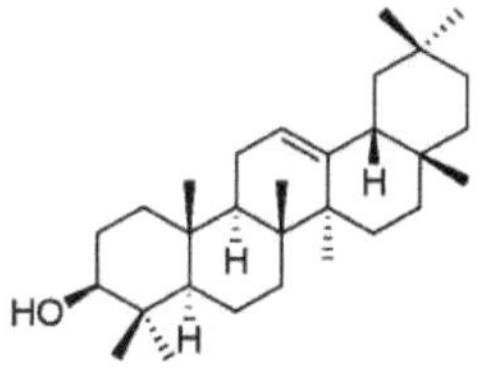

V

5.2 Identification of ursolic and oleanolic acids

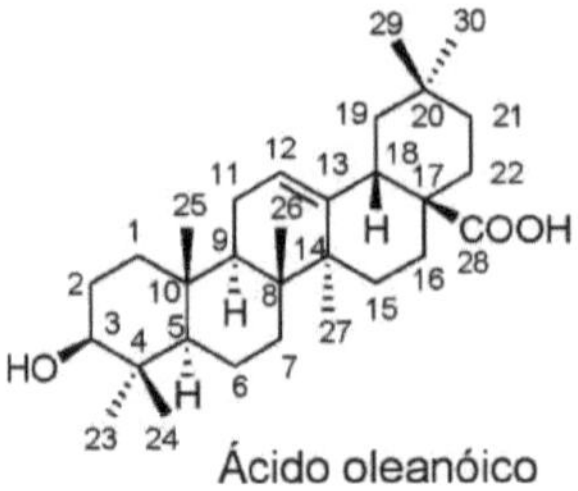

Ácido oleanóico 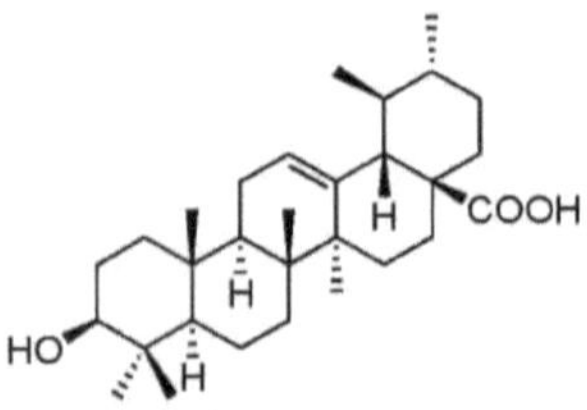 Ácido ursólico

When the melting point of ML-1 was obtained, it was observed that it had too wide a melting range to be attributed to a pure substance. The information obtained from the spectrum in the IR region, together with the information from the ^{1}H NMR and ^{13}C NMR spectra, suggests the presence of a triterpenoid. The IR spectrum of ML-1 (Appendix 7) shows an absorption band at 3460 cm^{-1} characteristic of O-H bond stretching. An intense absorption at 2942 cm^{-1}, characteristic of the stretching of C-H bonds of carbons with sp^2 hybridisation and an intense absorption band in the region of 1698 cm^{-1}, referring to the axial deformation of C=O bonds of saturated carboxylic acids. The multiple absorption bands between 1300 and 1000 cm^{-1} were attributed to the stretching of C-O bonds [119].

These data suggest the presence of carboxyl (-COOH) and possibly hydroxyl (-OH) groups in the structure of this substance.

The ^{1}H NMR spectrum (Annex 8) shows a profile typical of triterpene substances [120,121], which is basically characterised by the number and complexity of the signals between δ 0.5 and 2.0, referring to the methyl, methylenic and methinic groups common to the structure of compounds of this nature. The signal at *δ5*.20 (1 H, *sl)* corresponds to the hydrogen attached to carbon 12. The signal at *δ4*.30 is attributed to the hydrogen of the hydroxyl group at C-3, attached to H-3 [122]. The signal at *δ2*.99 corresponds to H-3, which, occupying an axial position, should give rise to a double duplet, with coupling constants around 10 and 5 Hz [122]. However, a more complex signal is observed due to coupling with the hydrogen of the OH group, which does not undergo chemical exchange due to interaction with the solvent [123].

The duplet at δ 2.10 (Appendix 9) corresponds to the hydrogen bonded to the C-18 in ursane and the double duplet at δ 2.75 corresponds to the hydrogen bonded to the C-18 in oleanane [120].

Analysing the chemical profile of Miconia reveals that most of the triterpenes isolated from species of the genus have oleanane and ursane structures, with the carboxyl group commonly present at position 28 [97,124]. The basic difference between these types of structures lies in the position in which the methyl group (C29) is attached, as can be seen in Figure 3.

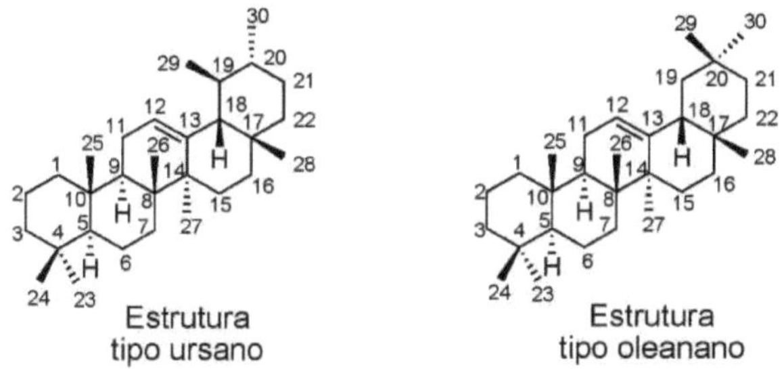

Figure 3 - Basic structure of ursane and oleanane triterpenes

These triterpene groups can be distinguished by the ^{13}C NMR of olefinic carbons 12 and 13, where C-12 is unprotected at around 2 ppm and C-13 is protected at around 5 ppm in the ursanes, compared to the corresponding olefinic carbons 12 and 13 in the oleanes [125].

The ^{13}C NMR spectrum of ML-1 (Appendix 10) shows pairs of signals at δ 124.9 -138.5 and δ 121.8 -144.1 referring to the C-12 and C-13 olefinic carbons that characterise the mixture of ursane and oleanane isomers. The signals at £77.1 and £72.0 are assigned to the C-3 carbinol carbons. At δ 178.9 and 178.6 there are signals from the carbonyl carbon at C-28 of both structures [126]. In order to corroborate the structural elucidation of ML-1, comparisons were made of the ^{13}C NMR signals of ML-1 (Table 6) with the data obtained in the literature for ursolic acid (ursane) and oleanoic acid (oleanane) [127].

Table 6 - ^{13}C NMR data of ML-1 compared to literature data for ursolic acid and oleanoic acid (400MHZ, DMSO-d6)

Carbon	ML-1 (ursane)	Ursolic acid[1]	ML-1 (oleanane)	Oleanoic acid[2]
1	38,7 (t)	38,9 (t)	38,7 (t)	38,9 (t)
2	23,6 (t)	23,5 (t)	27,8 (t)	27,9 (t)

3	77,1 (d)	78,3 (d)	72,0 (d)	78,0 (d)
4	36,9 (s)	37,3 (s)	38,7 (s)	39,3 (s)
5	55,1 (d)	55,7 (d)	55,1 (d)	55,7 (d)
6	18,3 (t)	18,7 (t)	18,3 (t)	18,7 (t)
7	33,0 (t)	33,3 (t)	33,0 (t)	33,3 (t)
8	38,7 (s)	39,3 (s)	38,7 (s)	39,8 (s)
9	45,7 (d)	46,7 (d)	47,1 (d)	47,9 (d)
10	36,9 (s)	37,2 (s)	37,0 (s)	37,2 (s)
11	23,7 (t)	23,8 (t)	23,7 (t)	23,8 (t)
12	124,9 (d)	125,5 (d)	121,8 (d)	122,3 (d)
13	138,5 (s)	139,2 (s)	144,1 (s)	144,3 (s)
14	41,9 (s)	42,0 (s)	41,9 (s)	42,0 (s)
15	28,5 (t)	28,4 (t)	28,5 (t)	28,4 (t)
16	23,1 (t)	22,7 (t)	24,1 (t)	23,8 (t)
17	47,1 (s)	47,9 (s)	45,6 (s)	46,6 (s)
18	52,7 (d)	53,4 (d)	41,9 (d)	42,0 (d)
19	38,7 (d)	39,3 (d)	45,6 (t)	46,6 (t)
20	38,7 (d)	39,8 (d)	30,7 (s)	30,9 (s)
21	30,7 (t)	30,9 (t)	33,0 (t)	33,5 (t)
22	36,9 (t)	37,3 (t)	33,0 (t)	33,3 (t)
23	28,6 (q)	28,6 (q)	28,6 (q)	28,6 (q)
24	16,4 (q)	16,5 (q)	16,4 (q)	16,5 (q)
25	15,6 (q)	15,6 (q)	15,6 (q)	15,6 (q)
26	16,4 (q)	16,5 (q)	17,3 (q)	17,5 (q)
27	23,6 (q)	23,5 (q)	25,9 (q)	26,0 (q)
28	178,9 (s)	179,8 (s)	178,6 (s)	179,8 (s)
29	17,3 (q)	17,3 (q)	33,0 (q)	33,3 (q)
30	21,4 (q)	21,3 (q)	24,1 (q)	23,8 (q)

[1,2] Data reported by JUNGES et al. [127] in $CDCl_3$.

Therefore, all the data obtained through the spectroscopic analyses of the isolated substance, as well as the comparison with data from the literature, allowed it to be identified as a mixture of 3β-hydroxyurs-12-en-28-oic acid (ursolic acid) and 3β-hydroxyolean-12-en-28-oic acid (oleanoic acid).

5.3. Identification of the acetylated product of ursolic acid

Confirmation that the product of the ursolic acid acetylation reaction had been obtained was made by comparison with the authentic standard using CCDC (mobile phase n-hexane/ethyl acetate (50:50) v/v, rf = 0.85).

5.4. Identification of the esterified product of ursolic acid

Confirmation that the product of the ursolic acid esterification reaction had been obtained was made by comparison with the authentic standard using CCDC (mobile phase n-hexane/ethyl acetate (50:50) v/v, rf = 0.80).

5.5. Identification of the salt derived from ursolic acid

The potassium salt derivative of ursolic acid was identified by positive cone electrospray mass spectrometry (appendix 11). The ion at m/z 495 corresponds to the protonated derivative $[M+H]^+$. The ions at m/z 517 and 533 correspond to the potassium salt derivative of ursolic acid cationised with sodium $[M+Na]^+$ and with potassium $[M+K]^+$, respectively.

5.6 Results of the antimicrobial activity evaluation

5.6.1 MIC results for the crude extracts of M. ligustroides

The MIC results for the crude extracts of M. ligustroides are shown in Table 7.

Table 7: Results of the minimum inhibitory concentration (MIC) in pg/mL for the crude extracts of *M. ligustroides* against the selected microorganisms.

	Extract n-hexane	Dichloromethane extract	Extract ethanol	Control (+)
BacilluscCereus (ATCC 14579)	375	625	475	Vanco: 0.18
Vibrio cholerae (ATCC 9458)	>1.000	>1.000	875	Genta: 0.73
Salmonella chleraesius (ATCC 10708)	>1.000	>1.000	>1.000	Genta: 0.36
Klebsiella pneumoniae (ATCC 10031)	>1.000	>1.000	425	Imip: 2.95
Klebsiella pneumoniae (ATCC 700603)	>1.000	>1.000	>1.000	Imip: 2.95
Pseudomonas aeruginosa	>1.000	>1.000	>1.000	Imip: >5.90
Escherichia coli	>1.000	>1.000	>1.000	Imip: 2.95
Enterococcus faecalis	375	>1.000	>1.000	Vanco: 0.18
Staphylococcus aureus	>1.000	>1.000	>1.000	Vanco: 0.18
Streptococcus pneumoniae (ATCC 6305)	450	475	375	Vanco: 0.18

* Vanco: Vancomycin; Genta: gentamicin; Imip: Imipenem.

The crude extracts showed low activity against the selected microorganisms. The best activities were obtained against the microorganisms B. cereus and S. peneumoniae. For the microorganisms K. pneumonieae (ATCC 10031) and E. faecalis, the extracts in ethanol and n-hexane were the most active, respectively.

5.6.2 MIC results for substances isolated from M. ligustroides

The substances isolated from M. ligustroides were evaluated in antimicrobial activity tests. The MIC results are shown in Table 9. Figure 4 shows the chemical structures of the substances evaluated. The best results were obtained for ursolic and oleanolic acids against the microorganism B. cereus. It should also be noted that for this microorganism the mixture of the two acids did not potentiate the antimicrobial effect. Oleanolic acid also showed considerable results against the microorganisms E. faecalis and S. pneumoniae. The substance β-sitosterol showed no activity against the selected microorganisms

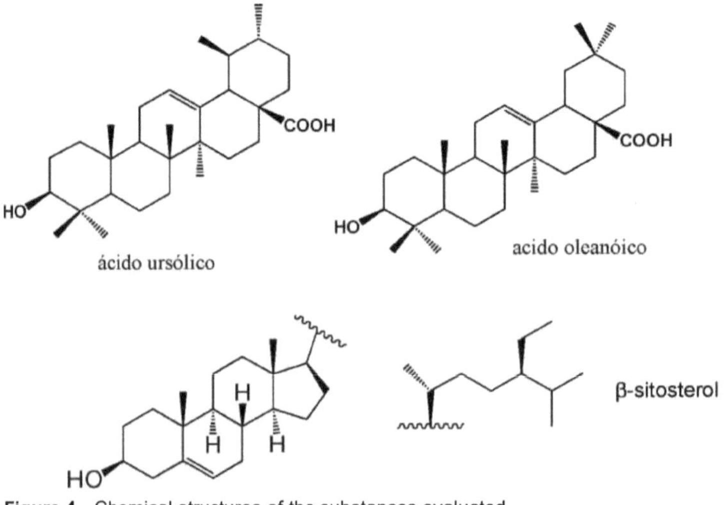

Figure 4 - Chemical structures of the substances evaluated

Table 8 - MIC results in pg/mL for the substances isolated from *M. ligustroides*.

	Mixing AU+AO	Acid Ursolic	Acid Oleanolic	-Sitosterol
Bacillus cereus (ATCC 14579)	> 1000	20	80	>1.000
Vibrio cholerae (ATCC 9458)	1000	> 1000	> 1000	>1.000
Salmonella chleraesius (ATCC 10708)	1000	> 1000	> 1000	>1.000
Klebsiella pneumoniae (ATCC 10031)	1000	> 1000	> 1000	>1.000
Klebsiella pneumoniae (ATCC 700603)	> 1000	> 1000	> 1000	>1.000
Pseudomonas aeruginosa	1000	> 1000	> 1000	>1.000

Escherichia coli	> 1000	> 1000	> 1000	>1.000
Enterococcus faecalis	> 1000	200	80	>1.000
Staphylococcus aureus	> 1000	> 1000	> 1000	>1.000
S. pneumoniae (ATCC 6305)	> 1000	> 1000	80	>1.000

* The positive controls are the same as those described in table 8.

5.6.3 MIC results for the semi-synthetic derivatives of ursolic acid.

Table 09 shows the results obtained for the MICs of the derivatives obtained from ursolic acid. In general, the derivatives obtained (Figure 5) did not respond in such a way as to reduce the MIC values against the selected microorganisms. The results were only optimised for S. pneumoniae, where all three derivatives were more active than ursolic acid. For the microorganisms Bacillus cereus and Enterococcus faecalis, the MIC results of the derivatives indicate a decrease in the inhibitory effect, leading to the conclusion that the hydroxyl (OH) and carbonyl (COOH) groups linked to carbons 3 and 17 in ursolic acid are important for the activity against these microorganisms.

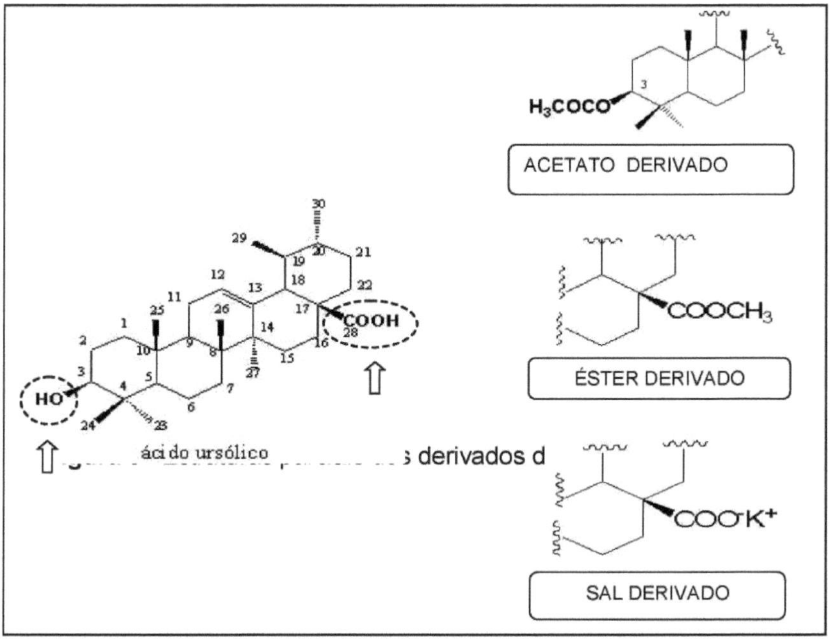

ACETATO DERIVADO

ÉSTER DERIVADO

SAL DERIVADO

Table 09: MIC results in pg/mL for ursolic acid derivatives.

	Acetylated	Ester	Salt	Acid Ursolic
Bacillus cereus (ATCC 14579)	>1.000	>1.000	> 1000	20
Vibrioccholerae (ATCC 9458)	>1.000	>1.000	> 1000	> 1000

Salmonella chleraesius (ATCC 10708)	>1.000	>1.000	> 1000	> 1000
Klebsiella pneumoniae (ATCC 10031)	>1.000	>1.000	> 1000	> 1000
Klebsiella pneumoniae (ATCC 700603)	>1.000	>1.000	> 1000	> 1000
Pseudomonas aeruginosa	>1.000	>1.000	> 1000	> 1000
Escherichia coli	>1.000	>1.000	> 1000	> 1000
Enterococcus faecalis	>1.000	>1.000	> 1000	200
Staphylococcus aureus	>1.000	>1.000	> 1000	> 1000
S. pneumoniae (ATCC 6305)	50	50	300	> 1000

* The positive controls are the same as those described in table 8.

CHAPTER 6

FINAL CONSIDERATIONS

According to the results obtained, it was possible to draw the following conclusions: 1. the crude extracts (n-hexane, dichloromethane and ethanol) obtained from M. ligustroides showed low activity against the microorganisms selected in this study. The best activities of the extracts were obtained against the microorganisms B. cereus and S. pneumoniae;

2. With regard to the isolated substances, the triterpenes ursolic acid and oleanolic acid showed the best results in terms of activity against B. cereus microorganisms. The mixture of these two substances was unable to potentiate the antimicrobial effect on this same microorganism. Oleanolic acid also showed a MIC below 100µg/mL against the microorganisms E. *faecales and S. pneumoniae. The* substance β-sitosterol showed no activity against the selected microorganisms;
3. In general, the semi-synthetic derivatives prepared from ursolic acid were unable to reduce the MIC values against the selected microorganisms.

The results were only optimised for the microorganism S. pneumoniae, where the three derivatives prepared were more active when compared to ursolic acid. For the microorganisms B. cereus and E. faecalis, the MIC results of the semi-synthetic derivatives indicated a reduction in the inhibitory effect, demonstrating that the hydroxyl (OH) and carboxyl (COOH) groups present in the chemical structure of ursolic acid are important for the activity against these microorganisms.

CHAPTER 7

BIBLIOGRAPHICAL REFERENCES

1. DI STASI, L. C. Plantas medicinais: arte e ciência um guia de estudo interdisciplinar. Editora UNESP, São Paulo, p.230, 1996.

2. CAETANO, N.; SARAIVA, A.; PEREIRA, R., CARVALHO. D., PIMENTEL, M. C. B,; MAIA, M. B. S. Determination of the antimicrobial activity of plant extracts popularly used as anti-inflammatory agents. Revista Brasileira de Farmacognosia, São Paulo, v. 12, supl., p. 132-135, 2002;

3. HOSTETTMANN, Kurt et al. Active principles of higher plants. Editora EdUFSCAR, São Carlos, p. 152, v. 4, 2003;

4. NEWMAN, D. J., GRAGG, G. M; SNADER, K. M. Natural Products as Sources of New Drugs over Period 1981-2002. J. Nat. Prod, v. 66, p. 1022-1037, 2003;

5. MONTANARI, C. A., BOLZANI, V. S. Rational drug planning based on natural products. Química Nova, São Paulo, v. 24, n.1. p. 105111, 2001;

6. ROBBERS, J. E., SPEEDIE, M. K., TYLER, V. E. Farmacognosia e Farmacobiotecnologia, São Paulo: Premier, 1997;
7. KOROLKOVAS, A. The potential richness of our flora. Revista Brasileira de Farmacognosia, São Paulo, v. 1, p. 1-7, jan./jun. 1996;

8. BORRIS, R. P. Natural products research: perspectives from a major pharmaceutical company. Journal of Ethnopharmacology, Limerick, v. 51, n. p. 29-38, Apr. 1996;

9. SIMÕES, C.M. O.; SCHENKEL, E. P.; GOSMANN, G.; MELLO, J. C. P.; MENTZ, L.A.; PETROVICK, P. R. **Farmacognosia: da planta ao medicamento**. Florianópolis/Porto Alegre: Ed. da UFSC, 1999;

10. WENIGER, B. Interest and limitation of a global ethnopharmacological survey. Journal of ethnopharmacology, Limerick, v.32, n. 1-3, p. 37-41, Apr. 1991;
11. DONATINI, R. S. Pharmacognostic and pharmacological study of Syzyum *jambos* (L.). **Dissertation (Master's Degree in Pharmacy)** - Faculty of Pharmaceutical Sciences, University of São Paulo, São Paulo. Alston, 95 f 2003;

12. CALIXTO, J. B. Biodiversity as a source of medicines Rev. Ciência e Cultura 3:37-39, 2003;

13. RENNER, S. S. Phylogeny and classification of the Melastomataceae and Memecylaceae Nord. J. Bot., v. 13, p. 519-540, 1993;
14. JOLY, A. B. Botany. Introduction to plant taxonomy. Editora da Universidade de São Paulo, São Paulo, p. 777, 1993;

15. WURDACK, J. J. & RENNER, S. S. Melastomataceae. In: Van Rijn (ed). Flora of the Guianas. Koeltz Scientific Books, Koenigstein, 1993;

16.MARTINS, A. B., SEMIR, J., GOLDENBERG, R. & MARTINS, E. The genus Miconia RUIZ & PAV. (Melastomataceae) in the state of São Paulo. Acta bot. bras. v. 10, p. 267-316, 1996;

17.COGNIAUX, A. Melastomataceae: In: A. & C. de Candolle (eds) Monographie Phanaerogamarum 7, G. Masson, Paris, 1891;

18.JUDD, W. S. Taxonomic studies in the Miconieae (Melastomataceae) Ann. Missouri Bot. Gard., v. 76, p. 476-495, 1989;

19.BAUMGRATZ, J. F. A. Myconias from the municipality of Rio de Janeiro. Section Miconia DC. (Melastomataceae). Rodriguésia, v. 32, p. 73-95, 1980;

20.BAUMGRATZ, J. F. A. Myconias of the State of Rio de Janeiro. Section Tamonea (Aibl.) Cogn. (Melastomataceae). Archos. Jard. Bot., v. 26, p. 6986, 1982;

21.BAUMGRATZ, J. F. A. Myconias from the municipality of Rio de Janeiro. Section Chaenanthera Naud. (Melastomataceae). Rodriguésia, v. 36, p. 45-58, 1984;

21.PEREIRA. E. Flora of the state of Guanabara IV. Melastomataceae II. Miconieae. Genus Miconia. Archos. Jard. Bot., v. 18, p. 183-214, 1964;

22.WURDACK, J. J. Melastomataceae of Santa Catarina. Sellowia, v. 14, p. 109-217, 1962;

23. WURDACK, J. J. Melastomataceae. In. T. Lasser (Ed) Flora de Venezuela, v. 8, Instituto Botanico, Caracas, 1973;

24. WURDACK, J. J. Melastomataceae. In G. Harling & b. Sparre (Eds) *Flora of Ecuador, v.* 13, University Goteborg and Risksmuseum, Stockholm, 1980;

26. PRICE, k. R. JOHNSON, I. T., FENWICK, G. R. The chemistry and biological significance of saponins in foods and feedingstuffs, *CRC Crit. Food. Sci. Nutr.* v. 26, p. 27-135, 1987;

27. WANG, B. and JIANG, Z. H. Studies on oleanoic acid, Chin. *Pharm. J.* v. 27, p. 393-397, 1992;

28. NOVOTNY, L., VACHALKAOVA, A., BIGGS, D. Ursolic acid: An anti-tumorigenic and chemopreventive activity, *Neoplasma*. v. 48, p. 241-246, 2001;

29. LIU, J. Oleanoic acid and ursolic acid: research perspectives, *J. Ethnopharmacol.* v. 100, p. 92-94, 2005;

30. JEONG, H. G., KIM, H. G.,HWANG, Y. P. Involvement of cytokines in the hepatic expression of metallothionein by ursolic acid, Toxicol. Lett. v. 155(3), p. 369-76, 2005;

31. MICELI, N., TAVIANO, M. F., GIUFFRIDA, D., TROVATO, A., TZAKOU, O., GALATI, E. M. Anti-inflammatory activity of extract and fractions from Nepeta sibthorpii Bentham, J. Ethnopharmacol. v. 97, p. 261-266, 2005;

32. OVESNA, Z., VACHALKOVA, A., HORVATHOVA, K., TOTHOVA, D. Pentacyclic triterpenoic acids: new chemoprotective compounds, Minireview, Neoplasma, v. 51, p. 327-333, 2004;

33.FAVEL, A., STEINMETZ, M. D., REGLI, P., VIDAL-OLLIVIER, E., ELIAS, R. AND BALANSARD. G. In vitro antifungal activity of triterpenoid saponins. Planta Med. v. 60, p. 50-53, (1994).

34.LIU, J. Oleanolic acid and ursolic acid: research perspectives, J. Ethnopharmacol. v. 49, p. 57-68, 1995;

35.SZUSTER-CIESIELSKA, A., KANDEFER-SZERSZEN, M. Protective effects of betulin and betulinic acid against ethanol-induced cytotoxicity in HepG2 cells, Pharmacol. Rep. v. 57, p. 588-595, 2005;

36.KIM, N.Y., LEE, M.K., PARK, M. J., KIM, S. J.,PARK, H. J., CHOI, J. W., KIM, S. H., CHO, S. Y., LEE, J. S. Momordin Ic and oleanoic acid from Kochiae Fructus reduce carbon tetrachloride-induced hepatotoxicity in rats, J Med Food. v. 8, p. 177-183, 2005;

37.CHEN, Y., LIU, J., YANG, X., XU, H. Oleanoic acid nanosuspensions: preparation, in-vitro characterisation and enhanced hepatoprotective effect, J. Pharm. Pharmacol. v. 57, p. 259-264, 2005;

38.GUPTA, M. B., BHALLA, T. N., GUPTA, G. P., MITRA, C. R., BHARGAVA, K. P. Anti-inflammatory activity of natural products (I) Triterpenoids, Eur. J. Pharmacol. v. 6, p. 67-70, 1969;

39.TAKAGI, K. E. H., KATO, H. Anti-inflammatory activities of hederagenin and crude saponin isolated from Sapindus mukorossi Gaertn, Chem. Pharm. Bull. v. 28, p. 1183-1188, 1980;

40.DAI, Y., HANG, B. Q., TAN, L. W. Anti-inflammatory effect oleanoic acid, Chinese J. Pharm. Toxicol. v. 3, p. 96-99, 1989;

41. SINGH, G. B., SINGH, S., BANI, S., GUPTA, B. D., BANERJEE, S. K. Anti-inflammatory activity of oleanoic acid in rats and mice, J. Pharm. Pharmacol. v. 44, p. 456-458, 1992;

42. DAI, Y., HANG, B. Q., MENG, Q. Y., MA, S. P., TAN, L. W. Inhibition of hypersensitivity reactions by oleanoic acid, Acta. Pharmacol. Sin. v. 9, p. 562565, 1988;

43. TSURUGA, T.,CHUN, Y. T., EBIZUKA, Y., SANKAWA, U. Biologically active constituents of Malaleuca leucadendron: inhibitors of induced histamine release from rat mast cells, Chem. Pharm. Bull. v. 39, p. 3276-3278, 1991;

44. NAJID, A., SIMON, A., COOK, J., CHABLE-RABINOVITCH, J. H., DELAGE, C., CHULIA, A., RIGAUD, J. M. Characterisation of ursolic acid as a

lipoxygenase and cyclooxygenase inhibitor using macrophages, platelets and differentiated HL 60 leukemic cells, Fed. Eur. Biochem. Soc. v. 299, p. 213217, 1992;

45. SIMON, A., NAJID, A., CHULIA, A. J., DELAGE, C., RIGAUD, M. Inhibition of lipoxygenase activity and HL60 leukemic cell proliferation by ursolic acid isolated from heather flowers (Calluna vulgaris), Biochim. Biophys. Acta. v. 1125, p. 68-72, 1992;

46. YING, Q.L., RNEHART, A. R., SIMON, S. R., CHERONIS, J. C. Inhibition of human leucocyte elastase by ursolic acid, Biochem. J. v. 277, p. 521-526, 1991;

47. ZHOU, C., SUN, X., LIU, W., SHI, H., GAO, H., MIAO, Y. Effects of oleanoic acid on the immune complex allergic reaction and inflammation, J. Clin.

Pharmacol. Sci. v. 2, p. 69-79, 1993;

48. GUPTA, M. B., NATH, R., GUPTA, G. P., BHARGAVA, K. P.Antiulcer activity of some plant triterpenoids, Indian J. Med. Res. v. 73, p. 649-52, 1981;

49. WRZECIONO, U., MALECKI, I., BUDZIANOWSKI, J., JIERYLOWICZ, H., ZAPRUTKO, L., BEIMVIK, E., KOSTEPSKA, H. Nitrogenous triterpene derivatives. Part 10: Hemisuccunates of some derivatives of oleanoic acid and their antiulcer effects, Pharmazie. v. 40, p. 542-544, 1985;

50. NGOUELA, S., NDJAKOU, B. L., TCHAMO, D. N., ZELEFACK, F., TSAMO, E., CONNOLLY, J. D. A prenylated xanthone with antimicrobial activity from the seeds of Symphonia globulifera, Nat. Prod. Res. v. 19, p. 23-27, 2005;

51. POEHLAND, B. L., CARTEF, B. K., RANCIS, T. A., HYLAND, L. J., ALLAUDEEN, H. S., TROUPE, N. In vitro antiviral activity of dammar resin triterpenes*, J. Nat, Prod.* v.50, p.706 - 713, 1987;

52. LIU, J., CHEN, X. F., XIA, L., GENG, X. Z., LI, Z. S. Effect of oleanoic acid on serum glyceride cholesterol and p-lipo-proteins in normal and experimental hyperlipidermic rats, *Chem. Pharm. Bull.* v. 4, p. 14-15, 1987;

53. MA, B. L. Hypolipidemic effects of oleanoic acid, Trad. *Med. Pharmacol*. v. 2, p. 28-29, 1986;

54. STEELE, J. C., WARHURST, D. C., KIRBY, G. C., SIMMONDS. M. S. In vitro and in vivo evaluation of betulinic acid as an antimalarial, *Phytother Res*. v. 13, p. 115-119, 1999;

55.TAKETA, A. T., GNOATTO, S. C., GOSMANN, G., PIRE, V. S., SCHENKEL, E. P., GUILLAUME, D. Triterpenoids from Brazilian Ilex species and their in vitro antitrypanosomal activity, *J. Nat. Prod.* v. 67, p. 1697-1700, 2004;

56.TORRES-SANTOS, E. C., LOPES, D., OLIVEIRA, R. R., CARAUTA, J. P., FALCAO, C. A., KAPLAN, M. A., ROSSI-BERGMANN, B. Antileishimanial activity of isolated triterpenoids from Pourouma guianensis, *Phytomedicine*. v. 11, p.114-120, 2004;

57.WANG, Q., FAN, M., BIAN, Z., NIE, M., CHEN, Z. Extract and identify ingredient from Ligustrum Lucidum Ait and study its effect to periodontal pathogen. Zhonghua Kou Qiang Yi Xue Za Zhi. v. 37(5), p. 388-390, 2002;

58.GUA, J. Q., WANG, Y., FRANZBLAU, S. G., MONTENEGRO, G., TIMMERMANN, B. N. Constituents of Quinchamalium majus with potential antitubercular activity, Z. Naturforsch., C, J. Biosci. v. 59, p. 797-802, 2004;

59.CHATTOPADHYAY, D., DUNGDUNG, S. R., MANDAL, A . B., MAJUMDER, G C. A potent sperm motility-inhibiting activity of bioflavonoids from an ethnomedicine of Onge, Alstonia macrophylla Wall ex A. DC, leaf extract, Contraception. v. 71, p. 372-378, 2005;

60.XU, L. Z., WAN, Z. X. The effect of oleanoic acid on acute hepatitis (70 cases), Humane Med. v. 7, p. 50-52, 1980;

61.MIZUSHINA, Y., ILDA, A., OTHA, K., SUGAWARA, F., SAKAGUCHI, K. Novel triterpenoids inhibit both DNA polymerase and DNA topoisomerase, Biochem J. v. 350, p. 757-763, 2000;

62.SYROVETS, T., BUCHELE, B., GEDIG, E., SLUPSKY, J. R., SIMMET, T. Acetyl-boswellic acids are novel catalytic inhibitors of human topoisomerases I and II alpha, Mol. Pharmacol. v. 58, p. 71-81, 2000;

63.DORAI, T., AGGARWAL, B. B., Role of chemopreventive agents in cancer therapy, Cancer Lett. v. 215, p. 129-140, 2004;

64.FU, L., ZHANG, S., LI, N., WANG, J., ZHAO, M., SAKAI, J., HASEGAWA, T., MITSUI, KATAOKA, T., OKA, T. S., KIUCHI, M., HIROSE, K., ANDO, M. Three new triterpenes from Nerium oleander and biological activity of the isolated compounds,J Nat. Prod. v. 68, p.198-206, 2005;

65.HUANG, M. T., HO, C. T., WANG, Z. Y., FERRARO, T.,LOU, Y. R., STAUBER, K., MA, W., GEORGIADIS, C., LASKIN, J. D., CONNEY, A. H. Inhibition of skin tumourigenesis by rosemary and its constituents carnosol and ursolic acid, Cancer, Res. v. 54, p. 701-708, 1994;

66.LEE, H. Y., CHUNG, H. Y., KIM, K. H., LEE, J. J. AND KIM, K. W. Induction of differentiation in the cultured F9 teratocarcinoma stem cells, Jpn. J. Clin. Oncol. v. 120, p. 513-518, 1994;

67.KONOPLEVA, M., TSAO, T., ESTROV, Z., LEE, R. M., WANG, R. Y., JACLSON, C. E., MCQUEEN, T., MONACO, G., MUNSELL, M., BELMONT, J., KANTARJIAN, H., SPORN, M. B., ANDREEFF, M. The synthetic triterpenoid 2-cyano-3,12-dioxooleana-1 9-dien-28-oic acid induces caspase- dependent and -independent apoptosis in acute myelogenous leukaemia, Cancer Res. v. 64, p. 7927-7935, 2004;

68.JIWAJINDA, S., SANTISOPASRI, V., MURAKAMI, A., KIM, O K., KIM, H. W., OHIGASHI, H. Suppressive effects of edible that plants on superoxide and nitric oxide generation, Asian Paci. J. Cancer Prev. v. 3, p. 215-223, 2002;

69.AGGARWAL, B.B., TAKADA, Y., OOMMEN, O. V. From chemoprevention to chemotherapy: common targets and common goals, Expert. Opin. Investig. Drugs v. 13, p. 1327-1338, 2004;

70.DIAZ, A. M., ABAD, M. J., FERNANDEZ, L., RECUERO, C., VILLAESCUSA, L., SILVAN, A M., BERMEJO, P. In vitro anti-inflammatory activity of iridoids and triterpenoid compounds isolated from Phillyrea latifolia, Biol. Pharm. Bull. v. 23, p. 1307-1313, 2002;

71.ACHIWA, Y., HASEGAWA, K., KOMIYA, T., UDAGAWA, Y. Ursolic acid induces Bax-dependent apoptosis through the caspase-3 pathway in endometrial cancer SNG-II cells, Oncol. Rep. v. 13, p. 51-57, 2005;

72.CÁRDENAS, C., QUESADA, A. R., MEDINA, M. A. Effects of ursolic acid on different steps of the angiogenic process, Biochem. Biophys. Res. Commun. v. 320, p. 402-408, 2004;

73.MUTO, Y., NINOMIYA, M., FUJIKI, H. Present status research on cancer chemoprevention in Japan, Jp. J. Clin. Oncol. v. 20, p. 219-224, 1990;

74.CUNHA, W. R., MARTINS, C., FERREIRA, D. S., CROTTI, A. E. M., LOPES, N., ALBUQUERQUE, S. In vitro trypanocidal activity of triterpenes from Miconia species. **Planta Med.**, v.9, n.5, p.470-472, 2003;

75. TRABULSI, L. R. et al. Microbiologia. 3 ed. Belo Horizonte: Ateneu, 1999;

76. SILVA, C. H. P. M. Bacteriologia. Teresópolis: Eventos, 1999.

77. LOGAMAYO, E. N. Antimicrobial resistance in major pathogens of hospital-acquired pneumonia in Asian countries. Am J. Infect. Control 36(4): 101-8, 2008;

78. EMNI, Y. Guid/bies for treatment of Pseudomona in intensive core units. Infez. Med. Suppl 7-17, 2005;

79. GISKE, L. G., MONNET, D. L., CARS, P., CARMELI, Y. Clinical and economic impact of common multidrug-resistant gram-negative bacilli.... Antimicrob Agents Chemother. J2(3): 813-21, 2008;

80. HSIEH, Y. C., LEE, W. S., SHAO, P. L., CHANG, L. Y., HUANG, L. M. The transforming Streptococcus pneumoniae in the 21st century. Chang Gung Med J. 31(2): 117-24, 2008;

81. SCOTT, J. A., BROOKS, W. A., PEIRIS, J. S., HOLTTMAN, D., MULHOLLAN, E. K. PseudomonaS research to reduct child hood mortality in the developing world. J. Chin. Invest. 118(4): 1291-1300, 2008;

82. HAWKEY, P. M. The growing burden of antimicrobial resistance. J. Antimicrob Chemothen, 62, Suppl 1, 1-9, 2008;

83. VAN RIJEN, M. M.; KLUYTMANS, J. A. New approaches to prevention of staphylococcal infection in surgery. Review. Curr Opin Infect Dis, 21(4): 3804, 2008;

84. ABUBAKAR, I., IRVINE, L., ALDUS, C.F., WYATT, G. M., FORDHAM, R., SCHELENZ, S., SHEPSTONE, L., HOWE, A., PECK, M., HUNTER, P. R. A

systematic review of the clinical, public health and cost-effectiveness of rapid diagnostic tests for the detection and identification of bacterial intestinal pathogens in faeces and food.Health Technol. **Assess,** 11(36): 1-211, 2007;

85.VILLAS-BOAS, G.T., PERUCA, A. P., ARANTES, O. M. Biology and taxonomy of Bacillus cereus, Bacillus anthracis, and Bacillus thuringiensis. (Review). Can J. Microbiol 53(6): 673-87, 2007;

86.LOPES, A. L., CLEMENS, J. D. DEN, J., JODAR, L. Cholera vaccines for the developing world (Review). Hum Vacin. 4(12): 165-9, 2008;

87.FARUQUE, S. M., NAIR, G. B. Molecular ecology of toxigenic Vibrio cholerae. Microbial Immunol 46(2): 59-66, 2002;

88.MOHAMED, J. A.; HUANG, D. B. Biofilm formation by enterococci. (Review) J. Med. Microbial 56, 1581-8, 2007;

89.RIBOULET E, VERNEUIL N, L A CARBONA S, SAUVAGEOT N, AUFFRAY Y, HARTKE A, GIARD J. C. Relationships between oxidative stress response and virulence in Enterococcus faecalis. J. Med. Microbial Biotechnol 13(1- 3): 140-6, 2007;

90.DE CHOMBRUN, P. G., COLOMBEL, J. F., POULAIN, D., DARFEVILLE-MICHAND, A. Pathogenic agents in inflammatory bowel diseases. Curr. Opin Gastroenterol, 24(4): 440-7, 2008;

91.FOLEY, S. L., LYNNE, A. M., NAYAK, R. Salmonella challenges: prevalence in swine and poultry and potential pathogenicity of sush isolates. J.Anim Sci. 2008 Apr; 86 (14 Suppl): E149-62. Epub Oct 2, 2007;

92.CALLAWAY, T. R., EDRINGTON, T.S., ANDERSON, RC, BYRD, J.A., NISBET, D.J. Gastrointestinal microbial ecology and the safety of our food

supply as related to Salmonella. J.Anim Sci. 2008 Apr; 86 (14 Suppl): E163- 72. Epub Sep 18, 2007;

93.CHIU, C.H., SU, L. H., CHU, C. Salmonella enterica serotype cholrraesuis: epidemiology, pathogenesis, clinical disease, and treatment. Clin. Microbiol Rev. Apr; 17(2): 311-22, 2004;

94.CHIU, C.H.; SU, L.H.; CHU, C. Salmonella enterica serotype choleraesuis: Epidemiology, Pathogenesis, Clinical Disease, and treatment. Clinical Microbiology Reviews, Apr. p. 311-322, 2004;

95.LOWRI ,J.B. The distribution and potential taxonomic value of alkylated ellagic acids. **Phytochemistry.** v. 7, p.1803-13, 1968;

96.MACARI, P. A. T., EMERENCIANO, V. P., FERREIRA ,Z. M. G. S. Identification of triterpenes from Miconia albicans Triana by microcomputer analysis. Quím. Nova, v.13(4), p. 260-262, 1990;

97.CHAN, W. R. SHEPPARD, U., MEDFORD, K. A., TINTO, W. F., REINOLDS, W. F., McLEANS, S. Triterpenes from Miconia stenostachya. J. Nat. Prod., v. 55, n. 7, p. 963-966, 1992;

98.GOLGHER, A. B., DE OLIVEIRA, A. B., RASLAN ,D. S., INTO, C. O. B. M. "Chemical study of *Miconia macrothirsa'.* an ecological approach" (Abstracts PN-40). 17ª *Annual Meeting of the Brazilian Chemical Society,* Caxambu, MG, 24 to

27 May 1994;

99. LI, X. C., JACOB, M. R., PASCO, D. S., ELSOHLY, H. N., NIMROD, A. C., WALKER, L. A., CLARK, A. M. Phenolic Compounds from Miconia myriantha Inhibiting Candida asartic Proteases. **J. Nat. Prod,** v. 64, p. 1282-1285, 2001;

100. HASRAT, J. A., DE BACKER, J. P., VAUQUEUM, G., VLIETINCK, A. J. Medicinal plants in Suriname: screening of plant extracts for receptorbinding activity. Phytomedicine, v. 4, p. 56-65, 1997;

101. LIMA, O. G., MARINI-BETOLLO, G. B., DELLE-MONACHE, F., COELHO, J. S. B., D'ALBUQUERQUE, J. L., MACIEL , J. M., LACERDA, A. L., MARTIUS, D. G. Antimicrobial and antineoplastic activity of a product identified as 2-methoxy-6-n-pentyl-p-benzoquinone (Primina) isolated from the roots of Miconia sp (Melastomataceae). Rev. Inst. Antibiot., Univ. Fed. Pernambuco, v. 10, p.29, 1970;

102. MARINI-BETOLO, G. B., DELLE MONACHE, F., GONÇALVES DE LIMA, O., BARROS COELHO, S. Miconidin, a new hydroquinone from the wood of Miconia sp (Melastomataceae). Gazz. Chim. Ital., v. 101, p.41-46, 1971;

103. GUNATILAKA, L. A. A., BERGER, N. J., EVANS, R., MILLER, J. S., WISSE, J. H., NEDDERMANN, K. M., BURSUKER, I., KINGSTON, D. G. Isolation, Synthesis, and Structure-Activity Relationships of Bioactive Benzoquinones from Miconia lepidota from the Suriname Rainforest. **J. Nat. Prod,** v. 64, p. 25, 2001;

104. ANTOUN, M. D., GERENA, L.; MILHOUS, W. K. Screening of flora of

Puerto Rico for potential antimalarial bioatives. Int. J. Pharmacog, v. 31, p. 255-58, 1993;

105. VASCONCELOS, M. A., FERREIRA, D. S., SILVA, M. L. A., VENEZIANI, R. C. S., CUNHA, W. R. Analgesic effects of crude extracts of Miconia albicans (Melastomataceae). Bollettino Chimico Farmacêutico, v. 142, n. 8, p. 333335, 2003;

106. CUNHA, W. R., VASCONCELOS, M. A., ROYO, V. A., FERREIRA, D. S., In vivo Analgesic and Anti-inflammatory Activities of Ursolic and Oleanoic Acid from *Miconia albicans* (Melastomataceae). Zeitschrift Fur Naturforschung C-A. **Journal of Biosciences,** v. 61, n. 7/8, p. 477-482, 2006;

107. ANDRADE E SILVA, M. L., CUNHA, W.R., PEDRO, C., GARCIA, P. A., MARTINS, C. Evaluation of the analgesic activity of an ethanol extract of *Miconia fallax*. *Bolletino Chimico Farmacêutico*, v. 141(2), p. 158-60, 2002;

108. ANDRADE E SILVA, M. L., CUNHA, W.R., PEDRO, C., GARCIA, P. A., MARTINS, C. Evaluation of the analgesic activity of an ethanol extract of *Miconia fallax*. Bolletino Chimico Farmacêutico, v. 141(2), p. 158-60, 2002;

109. RESENDE. F. A.; BARCALA, C. A. M. A.; FARIA, M. C. S.; KATO, F. H.; CUNHA, W. R.; TAVARES. D. C. Antimutagenicity of ursolic and oleanolic acid against doxorubicin-induced clastogenesis in Balb/c mice. Life Sciences 79, 1268-1273, 2006;

110. CUNHA, W. R., SILVA, M. L. A., TURATTI, I. C. C., FERREIRA, D. S., BETARELLO, H. L. Evaluation of the analgesic activity of *Miconia ligustroides* (Melastomataceae) using the abdominal writhing test in mice. Revista Brasileira de

Farmácia, v. 84, n. 2, p. 47-49, 2003;

111. SPESSOTO, M. A., FERREIRA, D. S., CROTTI, A. E. M, SILVA, M. L., CUNHA, W. R. Evaluation of the analgesic of extracts of Miconia rubiginosa (melastomataceae). **Phytomedicine,** v. 10(6-7), p. 606-9, 2003;

112. CUNHA, L. C. S.; SILVA, L. A.; FURTADO, N. A. J.; VINÓIS, A. H. C.; MARTINS, C. H. G.; FILHO, A. S. AND CUNHA. W. R. Antibacterial Activity of Triterpene Acids and Semi-Synthetic Derivatives against Oral Pathogens. Z. Naturforsch. 62c, 668-672, 2007;

113. CELOTTO, A. C., NAZÁRIO, D. Z., SPESSOTO, M. A., MARTINS, C. H. G. CUNHA, W. R. Evaluation of the in vitro antimicribial activity of crude extracts of three Miconia epecies. J. v. 61, n. 7/8, p. 477-482, 2006. three Miconia species. Brazilian Journal of Microbiology, v. 34, p. 339-340, 2003;

114. LI, X. C., JOSHI, A. S. Et al. Fatty Acid Synthase Inhibitors Plants: Isolation, Structure Elucidation, and SAR Studies. J. Nat. Prod, v. 64, p. 1909-1914, 2002;

115. JULIANA, R., DANIELLE, C. M., DANIEL, R., GUILHERME, J. Z., LOURDES, C. S., Wagner, V., HÉRIDA, R. N. S. Antimicrobial Activity of Miconia Species (Melastomataceae). J. Med. Food 11(1): 120-126, 2008;

116. KASHIWADA, Y., NAGAU, T., HASHIMOTO, A., IKESHIRO, Y., OKABE, H., COSENTINO, L. M., LEE, K-H. Anti-AIDS agents 38. Anti-HIV activity of 3-O- acylursolic acid derivatives. J. Nat. Prod., v. 63, p. 1619-1622, 200;

117. NCCLS. Methods for Dilution Antimicrobial Susceptibility Tests for Bacteria That Grow Aerobically; Approved Satndard-Sixth Edition. NCCLS document M7-A6 (ISBN) 1-56238-486-4). NCCLS, 940 West Valley Road, Suite 1400, Wayne, Pennsylvania, 2003;

118. PALOMINO, J. C., MARTIN, A., CAMACHO, M., GUERRA, H., SWINGS, J., PORTAELS, S. Resazurin microtiter assay plate: simple and inexpensive method for detection of drug resistance in Mycobaterium tuberculosis. Antimicrobial Agents Chemotherapy, v.46, n. 8, p. 622-625, 2001;

119. CREWS, P., RODRIGUES, J., JASPARS, M. Organic structure analysis, Oxford University Press, 1988;

120. HONGQUAN, D., YOSHIHISA, T., MOMOTA, H., OHMOTO, Y., TAKI, T., JIA, Y., LI, D. Trterpenoids from tripteygium wilfordii. Phytochemistry, v. 53, p. 805-810, 2000;

121. LEITE, J. V. Phytochemical study of the leaves of A. Triplinervia. *Master's* dissertation - *Faculty of Pharmacy, Federal University of Minas Gerais*, Belo Horizonte, 1998;

122. SILVERSTEIN, R. M., WEBSTER, F. X. Spectrometric Identification of Organic Compounds. Translation by Paula Fernandes de Aguiar and Ricardo Bicca de Alencastro. Original title: *Spectrometric Identification of Organic Compounds.* 6ª ed, Rio de Janeiro: Guanabara Koogan, 2000;

123. MAILLARD, M., ADEWUNMI, C. O., HOSTETTMANN, K. A triterpene glycoside from the fruits of tetrapleura tetraptera. Phytochemistry, v. 31, p. 1321-

1323, 1992;

124. GOLGHER, A. B., DE OLIVEIRA, A. B., RASLAN, D. S., PINTO, C. O. B. M. Chemical study of Miconia macrothyrsa: an ecological approach (Abstracts PN-40). 17ª *Annual Meeting of the Brazilian Chemical Society,* Caxambu, MG, 24 to 27 May 1994;

125. MAHATO, S. B., KUNDU, A. P. ^{13}C NMR spectra of Pentacyclic triterpenoids - a compilation and some salient features. *Phytochemistry, v. 37* (6), p. 15171575, 1994;

126. OLEA, R. S. G., ROQUE, N. F. Analysis of triterpene mixtures by ^{13}C NMR. *Chem. Nova*, v. 13(4), p. 278-281, 1990;

127. JUNGES, M. J., FERNANDES, J. B., VIEIRA, P. C., FERNANDES, M. F. G. S., FILHO, E. R., FRUHAUF, M., BARANAMO, A. G. Ursanic and oleanic triterpenes isolated from the stem of Eugenia florida DC. *Revista de Pesquisa e Pós-Graduação*, Erechim, RS, v. 01, p. 13-30, 2000;

128. MAEDA, H.; MATSU-URA, S.; YAMAUCHI, Y. OHMORI, H. Resazurin as an electronic acceptor in glucose oxidase-catalysed oxidation of glucose. *Chemical Pharmaceutical bulletin,* v. 49, n. 5, p. 622-625, 2001.

ANNEXES

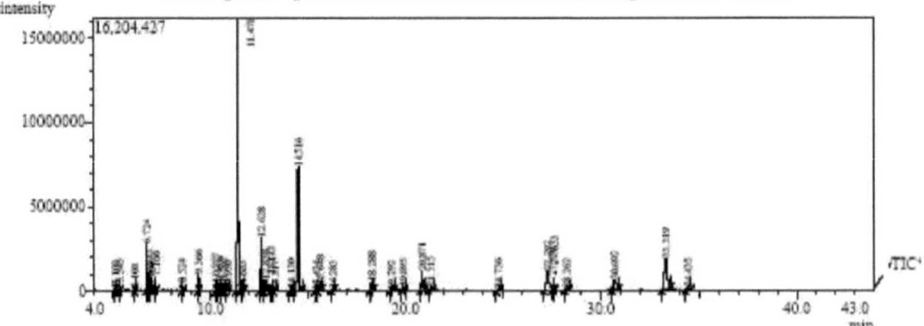

Peak Report TIC

Peak#	R.Time	Area	Area%	Name
1	5.108	479145	0.28	
2	5.345	563939	0.33	
3	6.108	123639	0.07	
4	6.724	3856638	2.24	
5	6.843	1038674	0.60	
6	6.960	116649	0.07	
7	7.166	99389	0.06	
8	8.524	706084	0.41	
9	9.366	1765598	1.03	
10	10.277	1161957	0.68	
11	10.476	695010	0.40	
12	10.707	827679	0.48	
13	10.930	164255	0.10	
14	11.478	59762851	34.74	
15	11.683	264039	0.15	
16	12.628	10709867	6.23	
17	12.838	2367906	1.38	
18	13.143	714423	0.42	
19	13.317	125802	0.07	
20	14.130	1205638	0.70	
21	14.516	32274386	18.76	
22	15.434	318670	0.19	
23	15.648	2459302	1.43	
24	16.283	436170	0.25	
25	18.288	2768097	1.61	
26	19.292	294269	0.17	
27	19.895	886614	0.52	
28	20.871	5825454	3.39	
29	21.315	1198736	0.70	
30	24.736	799871	0.46	
31	27.292	11431849	6.64	
32	27.550	13587	0.01	
33	27.633	10479	0.01	
34	28.262	710481	0.41	
35	30.692	5516210	3.21	
36	33.319	18759388	10.90	
37	34.435	1590404	0.92	
		172043149	100.00	

Annex 1: GC-MS chromatogram of the n-hexane **extract of** M. ligustroides

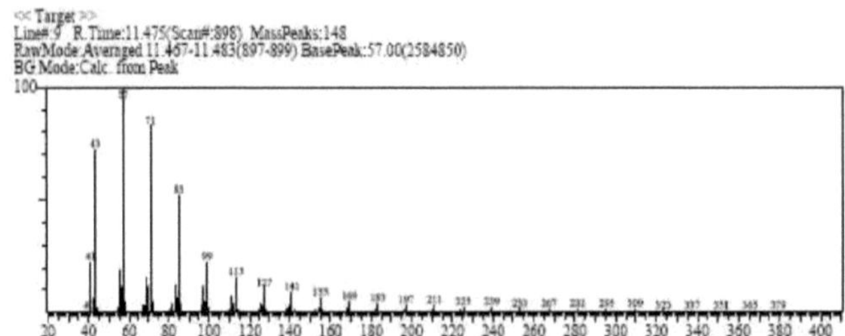

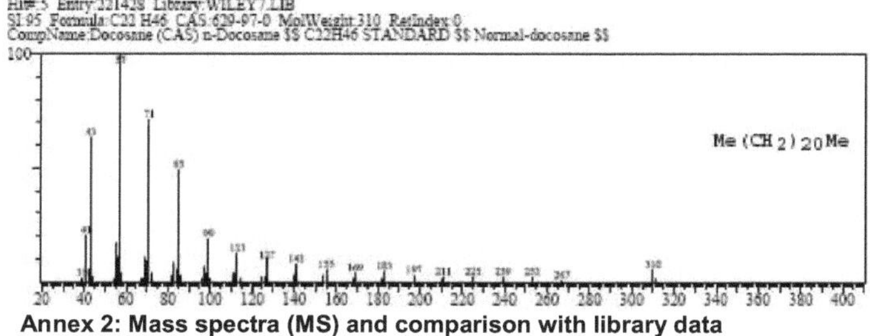

Annex 2: Mass spectra (MS) and comparison with library data

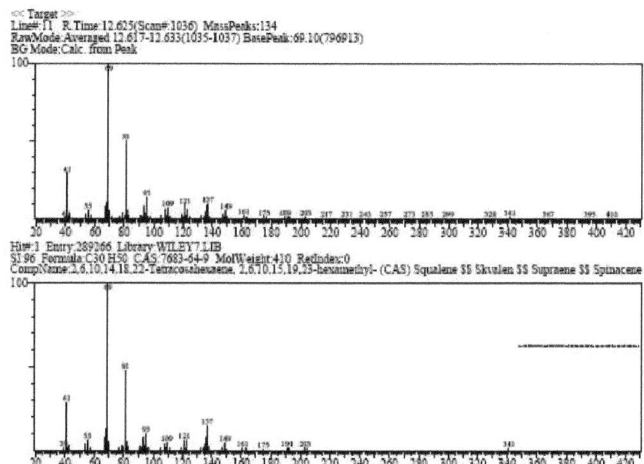

Annex 3: Analysis of the peaks obtained and comparison with library data

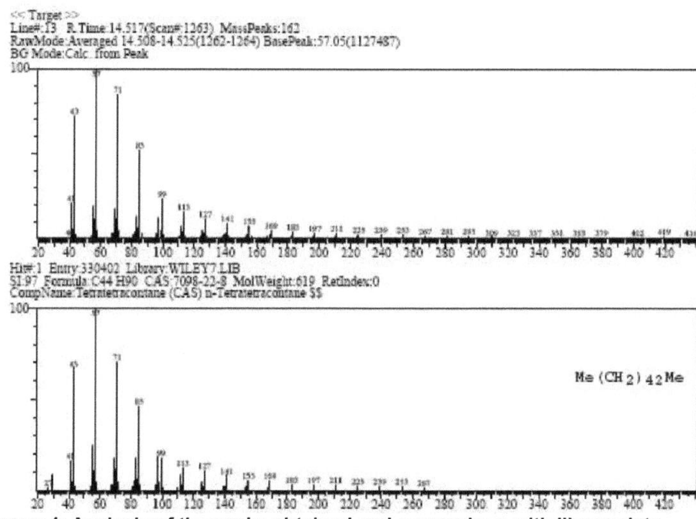

Annex 4: Analysis of the peaks obtained and comparison with library data

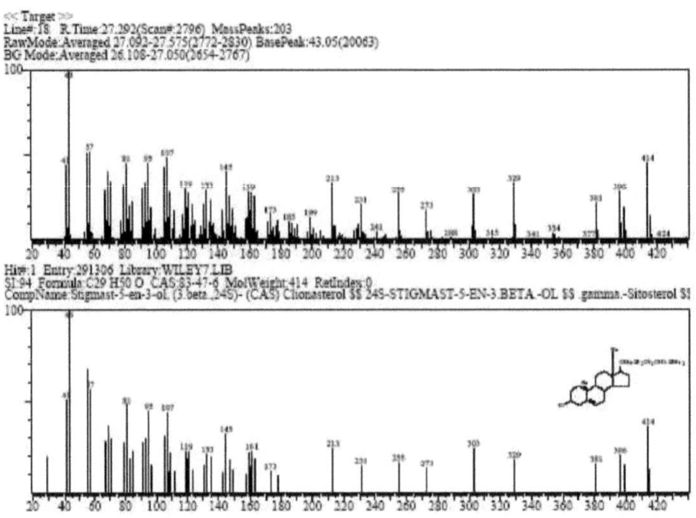

Annex 5: Analysis of the peaks obtained and comparison with library data

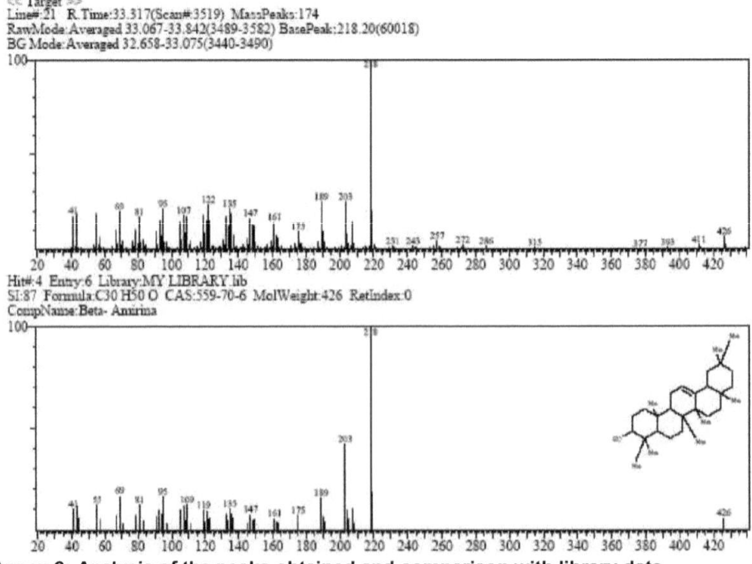

Annex 6: Analysis of the peaks obtained and comparison with library data

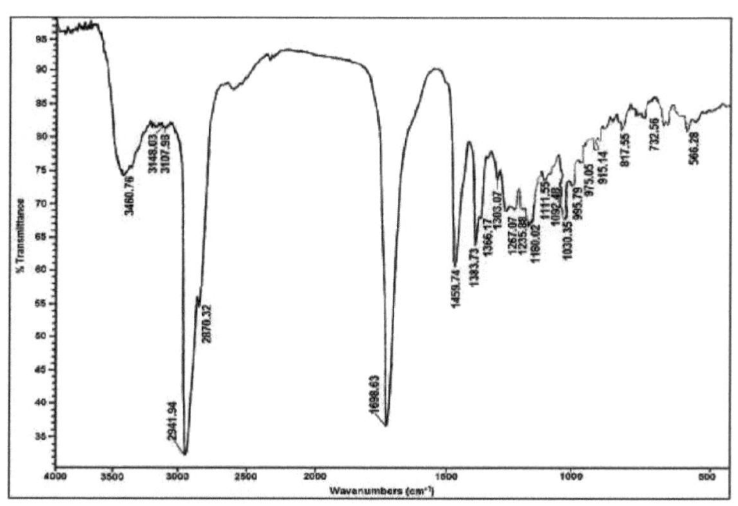

Annex 7: IR absorption spectrum of ML-1

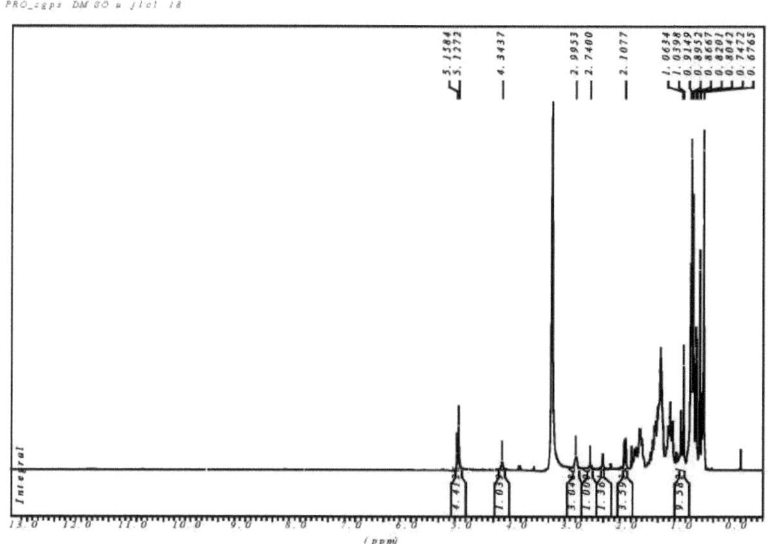

Annex 8: ^{1}H NMR spectrum (300 MHz, DMSO-d6) **of ML-1**

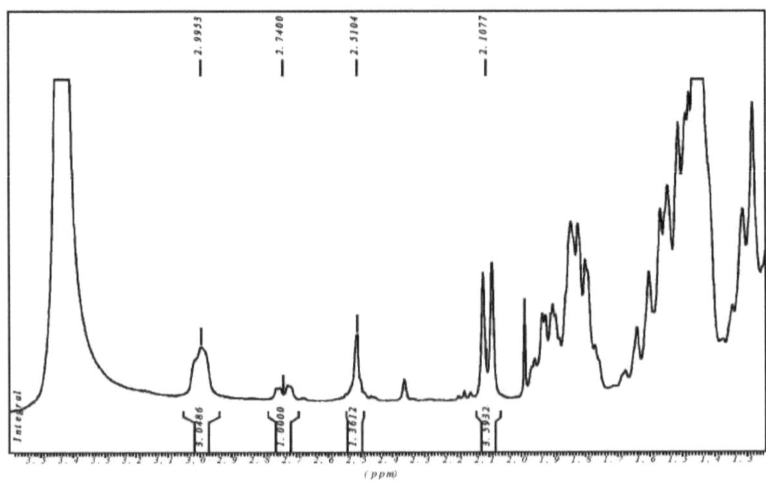

Annex 9: Expansion of the ^{1}H NMR spectrum of ML-1

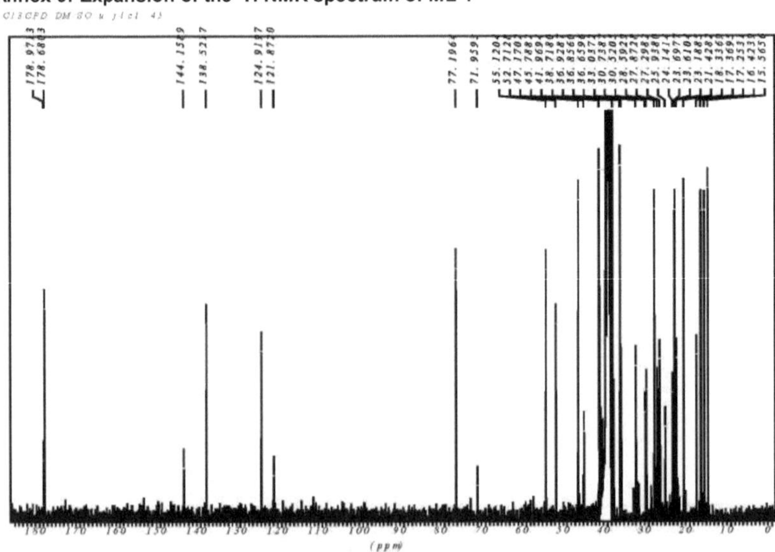

Annex 10: ^{13}C NMR spectrum (75 MHz, DMSO-d6**) of ML-1**

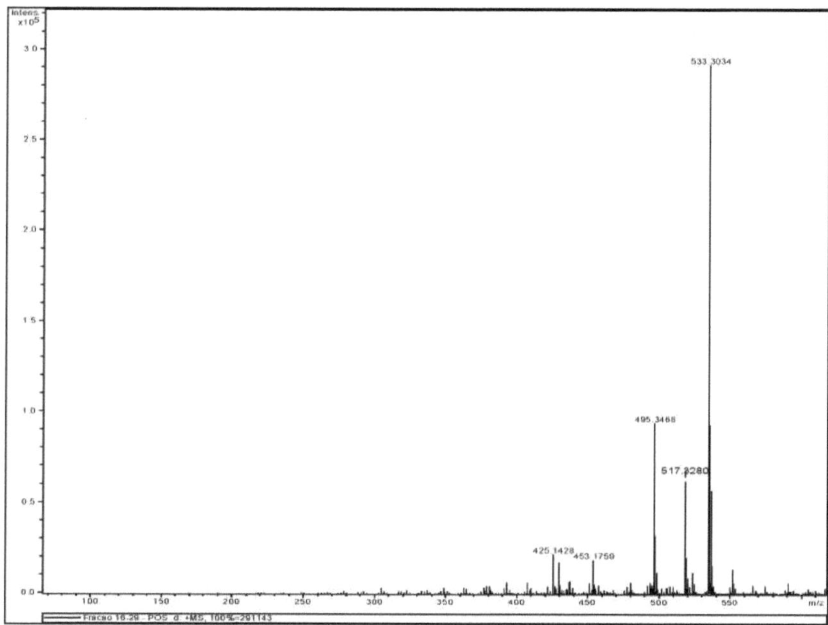

Annex 11: Mass spectrum (positive electrospray-cone) of the potassium salt of ursolic acid

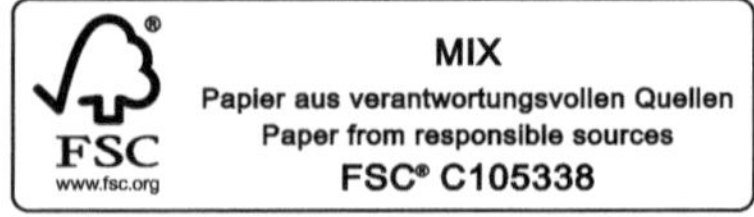

Printed by Books on Demand GmbH, Norderstedt / Germany